DR. ISADORE ROSENFELD'S
2005
BREAKTHROUGH
HEALTH

DR. ISADORE ROSENFELD'S
2005
BREAKTHROUGH
HEALTH

Up-to-the-Minute
Medical News
You Need to Know

ISADORE ROSENFELD, M.D.

RODALE®

Notice

This book is intended as a reference volume only, not as a medical manual. The information given here is designed to help you make informed decisions about your health. It is not intended as a substitute for any treatment that may have been prescribed by your doctor. If you suspect that you have a medical problem, we urge you to seek competent medical help.
Mention of specific companies, organizations, or authorities in this book does not imply endorsement by the author or publisher, nor does mention of specific companies, organizations, or authorities imply that they endorse this book, its author, or the publisher. Internet addresses and telephone numbers given in this book were accurate at the time it went to press.

Printed in the United States of America
Rodale Inc. makes every effort to use acid-free ∞, recycled paper ♲.

Book design by Drew Frantzen

ISBN-13 978–1–59486–140–6   paperback
ISBN-10 1–59486–140–4   paperback
ISBN-13 978–1–59486–191–8   hardcover
ISBN-10 1–59486–191–9   hardcover

Distributed to the trade by Holtzbrinck Publishers

2   4   6   8   10   9   7   5   3   1   paperback
2   4   6   8   10   9   7   5   3   1   hardcover

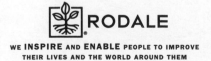

RODALE
WE **INSPIRE** AND **ENABLE** PEOPLE TO IMPROVE
THEIR LIVES AND THE WORLD AROUND THEM

FOR MORE OF OUR PRODUCTS
WWW.RODALESTORE.COM
(800) 848-4735

To my seven wonderful grandchildren,
the most important "breakthroughs" in my life.

CONTENTS

ACKNOWLEDGMENTS

NO BOOK, regardless of the author's ability and experience, can make it without a good editor. Editing a professional book, be it on architecture, engineering, or medicine, must be more difficult than editing a novel. In addition to the usual skills required, a lay editor must be able to interpret the special information to which the author is privy. My editor at Rodale, Leah Flickinger, has a knack for judging what's important and how best to present it. I appreciate her talent and input, although frankly, I am dismayed at the rumors that she now plans to practice medicine herself part-time.

Some 25 years ago, Joni Evans was the editor of my very first book. She went on to bigger and better things, such as becoming president of a publishing company. Currently she is one of the most sought-after book agents in New York. Still, she continues to check meticulously all my manuscripts with an editor's expertise, for which I thank her.

The hardest part of writing a book such as this is to verify its accuracy. Too often, statistics are misstated due to typos in the original source. I was very fortunate to have had Christina Bilheimer, Dana Ciccone, Kerry Holland, Meredith Pharaoh, and Deanna Portz assigned to check every single statement on every page. I know how arduous and time-consuming this was and want to express my gratitude to them.

Finally, nothing I write ever leaves my desk until my favorite wife, Camilla, has reviewed it. She has the most incredible judgment of anyone I know. If anything in this book bothers you, please call her, not me!

INTRODUCTION

THIS PAST YEAR, there have been innumerable advances in the prevention, diagnosis, and treatment of virtually every disease and disorder known to man. Some will stand the test of time, others will not. How does a patient make sense of all the conflicting health headlines? Which ones are real and promising? Which are hype?

To separate the wheat from the chaff, I have reviewed countless reports, read the most prestigious medical journals, and attended the most important medical meetings and conferences this past year. Most doctors do so to maintain their expertise, particularly in their own specialty. Some will share their new knowledge with you during an office visit; others will simply tell you about them when there is a need to do so. The truth is, unless you read this book, you may not hear about these findings at all.

I believe that it's important for you, the patient, to be aware of any research advances that may have an impact on your health. For example, if you have heart disease, you need to know that there are new target levels for the "bad" LDL cholesterol. If you have an enlarged prostate, you need to be aware that there is an easier and safer way to remove it—and a more effective treatment if that organ is cancerous. Such knowledge can enable you to contact your doctor immediately so you can derive the maximum possible benefit from medical progress before it's too late.

Last year's edition of *Breakthrough Health* is by no means outdated. *Breakthrough Health 2005* is meant to supplement it, not replace it. Most of the advances I reported last year have now become standard treatment and technically speaking are no longer "breakthroughs." However, in this volume, you'll learn which of last year's discoveries have not lived up to their expectations, in addition to what's new and important.

Here are just a few examples of the groundbreaking medical developments of the last 12 months.

- The statin drugs, originally prescribed to lower high cholesterol, have been found to be effective against a host of other diseases, ranging from cancer to osteoporosis.

- Regular commercial sunscreens may not protect you from all the sun's harmful rays. Read why—and what you can do about it.

- If you're taking the popular "natural" supplement melatonin to help you sleep, learn when *not* to do so.

- If you have the genes for breast cancer, read about new ways to prevent, diagnose, and treat this malignancy.

- It sounds almost too good to be true, but a common spice lowers blood sugar and cholesterol levels, and it's especially beneficial to people with diabetes (and anyone who is prone to it).

- There's a bottle in your medicine cabinet that contains what was once considered a potential lifesaver—but you should now get rid of it. Find out what it is and with what you should replace it.

- For years doctors have recommended vitamin E supplements. Should you be taking them if you have heart disease or are on a cholesterol-lowering statin drug? If not, why not?

- Coffee, milk, and wine can be both good *and* bad for you. Learn when they really help—or harm.

These are but a few of the exciting findings in *Breakthrough Health 2005*. Read it to stay up-to-date. Your life may depend on it.

ALLERGIES AND ASTHMA

• • • • • • • • •

When to Stay Away from Melatonin

MELATONIN, A HORMONE secreted by the pineal gland in the brain, regulates our internal clocks so that we sleep when we should and remain awake during the day. Melatonin production begins to increase in the evening before bedtime, and its concentration peaks in the middle of the night, enabling us to sleep. Just before we're due to wake up, its levels begin to fall, and then they taper off in the morning, helping us stay awake.

The brain makes less melatonin as we grow older, which may explain why some elderly men and women suffer from insomnia. (Interestingly enough, this observation has recently been challenged in one study that reports no difference in the levels of melatonin in young and elderly persons.) In response to these physiological observations, the ever-alert "health food" industry is promoting melatonin dietary supplements for the management of insomnia and jet lag. Its use is currently being evaluated in shift workers with changing schedules, as well as for controlling seizures, seasonal affective disorder (SAD), and depression. The usual adult dose of 1 to 3 milligrams a day is considered to be safe.

HERE'S WHAT'S NEW

Earlier studies have shown that melatonin releases chemicals that promote inflammation (nonsteroidal anti-inflammatory drugs, aspirin, and statin drugs reduce it). Researchers at the National Jewish Medical and Research Center in Denver measured the melatonin levels round the clock for 7 days in 7 people with asthma whose symptoms were worse at night, in 13 whose asthma attacks came on mostly during the day, and in 11 subjects without asthma. They found that although melatonin levels in all three groups were highest during the night, as one would expect, they were highest in people with asthma whose attacks were mostly nocturnal. According to the researchers, "these findings suggest that naturally produced melatonin increases inflammation in the airways and makes lung function worse." (This may explain why melatonin supplements appear to worsen sleep apnea, too.)

A recent small study suggests that taking 3 milligrams of melatonin before bedtime reduces the frequency, intensity, and duration of migraine headaches. The period of observation was only 3 minutes; a longer, more statistically significant trial is necessary. However, the protective effect of melatonin against migraine headaches has been suggested before. It may be worth trying it if your migraines are making you miserable.

THE BOTTOM LINE

If you have chronic asthma, especially the kind that's worse at night, you're better off taking something other than melatonin to help you sleep. However, if you have migraine headaches, 3 milligrams of melatonin at bedtime may make them more tolerable.

Inhaled Corticosteroid Safety

CORTICOSTEROIDS ARE POTENT DRUGS that reduce inflammation and mucus production in the airways of patients with asthma and chronic obstructive pulmonary disease. Serious side effects from their long-term oral use are much less common when they are inhaled. The four most commonly used agents in the United States for such inhalation therapy are Aerobid (flunisolide), Vanceril (beclometh), Azmacort (triamcinolone), and Pulmicort (budesonide).

There also has been uncertainty about the long-term effect of inhaled corticosteroids on bone health, since these medications may deplete or interfere with the absorption of calcium. That's because when a corticosteroid is inhaled, a small amount is actually swallowed and absorbed through the stomach into the body. Doctors have usually advised anyone who frequently uses this form of therapy to take calcium supplements.

The safety of using inhaled corticosteroids during pregnancy has also been questioned because of the suspicion that their use may result in low-birth-weight babies.

HERE'S WHAT'S NEW

The Second Expert Panel on Asthma (a national committee of experts representing 38 organizations specializing in asthma) states that "*inhaled* corticosteroids are the most effective long-term therapy available for mild, moderate, or severe persistent asthma." According to this panel, when taken in recommended doses, inhaled corticosteroids are safe, and they deliver potent anti-inflammatory therapy directly to the airways. Any adverse effects from these inhaled corticosteroids are far outweighed by the benefits.

After reviewing 14 major studies of patients on moderate to high doses of such therapy, researchers now believe that their long-term use does *not* have a significant effect on bone mineral density. These findings were reported at the Annual Scientific Assembly of the American College of Chest Physicians.

A recent study of almost 500 women, published in the *Journal of Allergy and Clinical Immunology* found that using inhaled steroids to treat persistent asthma during pregnancy does not harm the infant in any way. This should reassure women with asthma who require these medications while they are pregnant.

THE BOTTOM LINE

If you require inhaled corticosteroids for any reason, you may use them without fear of harming your bones and leaving you with osteoporosis or, if you're pregnant, of affecting your unborn child in any way. Still, I do suggest that those who require such therapy, especially women, take supplemental calcium.

Bleeding from Steroid Nasal Sprays

STEROID NASAL SPRAYS help allergy sufferers during the allergy season and do not carry the same risk as oral steroid medication. Most people use the right hand to spray in the right nostril and the left hand for the left nostril. Doing so directs the spray onto the nasal septum (the bone and cartilage that run down the middle of the nasal cavity), irritating it, eroding its lining, and because of its rich blood

supply, making it bleed. If this happens often enough, the spray must
be discontinued.

HERE'S WHAT'S NEW

The following practical observation by Talal Nsouli, M.D., reported to a meeting of the American College of Allergy, Asthma, and
Immunology, may not win him a Nobel Prize, but anyone plagued
with nosebleeds after repeated use of nasal steroid sprays will be
grateful to him. After testing 19 subjects with allergic rhinitis for 2
weeks, he found that using an alternate hand technique—the right
hand to spray in the left nostril and the left hand for the right nostril—aims the medication away from the septum and toward the
outer wall of the nose, dramatically reducing nosebleeds.

THE BOTTOM LINE

If you have allergic rhinitis and frequently use steroid sprays, your
chances of developing a nosebleed can be dramatically reduced by
switching hands when you spray into your nose. It's as simple as that.

ALZHEIMER'S
DISEASE
• • • • • • • • •

Recognize the Early Signs

WE HUMANS ARE VULNERABLE to many terrible afflictions, but in my experience, the one people fear most is Alzheimer's disease (AD). Losing the ability to think, to recognize, to interact, to belong, to continue relationships that you've enjoyed over a lifetime is devastating. This was dramatically demonstrated when the quality of life in President Reagan's last years was made public after his death. As many as 4 million Americans currently suffer from Alzheimer's disease, and some 12 to 15 million are expected to have it by the year 2050.

AD is a neurological disorder that strikes the areas of the brain primarily involved with thought, memory, and language. Most people wrongly believe that it is a manifestation of aging, which is why it was called senile dementia for so long. AD is not caused by aging; it's a disease, albeit one that happens to affect mostly older people. In fact, the German doctor who first described the disease characterized it as occurring not in the elderly but in middle-aged people!

The changes in the brain of someone with AD are very specific and quite different from those due to normal aging. AD is characterized by the presence of abnormal clumps, called amyloid plaques, as well as bundles of tangled nerves (neurofibrillary tangles) not found in the brains of normal older men and women. In this disease, nerve cells in parts of the brain that are critical to memory and thinking die. Decreased cognitive function in these patients may also be due to decreased amounts of certain chemicals that carry messages back and forth between nerve cells. These physical changes may not actually cause the symptoms of Alzheimer's; they may simply reflect its presence.

There is no cure for AD, but we are learning more and more about it every day.

Although there must be more than one contributing factor, age is the most important. AD is the seventh leading cause of death in those over 65—10 percent of whom already have the disease. The number of those afflicted doubles every 5 years thereafter. Half of Americans older than 85 probably have some degree of Alzheimer's. Family history is another risk factor. Several genes have been identified in some patients with AD. Their presence, however, does not ensure that AD will develop, and their absence is no guarantee that it won't.

AD usually develops gradually. Early on, the symptoms are only annoying, and life often continues more or less normally. But in time, the problem becomes apparent. These unfortunate men and women may lose the ability to think clearly, to understand, to read, to write, and, in short, to function normally. Many eventually need total care.

There is no single test to diagnose Alzheimer's with certainty during life, although positron-emission tomography (PET) scans of the brain do help by assessing its biochemical activity and revealing patterns of brain activity indicative of progressive dementia. They may also predict the course of the disease in patients with mild memory loss, language problems, and behavioral changes.

At the present time, however, the only sure way to diagnose Alzheimer's is after death—at autopsy.

Disturbing changes in behavior, especially among the elderly, are not always due to AD. There are other causes, the most common of which are multiple small strokes (usually the result of long-standing untreated high blood pressure) that have gone undiagnosed and ended up damaging areas of the brain dealing with cognition. On occasion, a brain tumor can also affect behavior, as can poor nutrition, notably vitamin B deficiency, especially in the elderly. That's why it's so important, when given the diagnosis of AD, to obtain a second opinion from a neurologist to make sure that some other cause, often treatable, isn't masquerading as Alzheimer's.

HERE'S WHAT'S NEW

The Alzheimer's Association recently prepared a checklist of the 10 most important warning signs of AD in order to help family members and health-care providers recognize the early onset of the disease.

Memory loss. Typical of AD is the tendency to forget recently learned information. Many of us do not recall appointments, names, telephone numbers, where we put our car keys, or exactly where in the huge parking lot we left our cars. If we're not concentrating or are distracted or preoccupied, such memory lapses are understandable and normal. But someone with Alzheimer's regularly forgets these "details."

Difficulty performing familiar tasks. People with AD are often unable to carry out everyday tasks that are performed almost automatically by most of us without our thinking about them. They may forget how to prepare a meal they have made for years, use a household appliance, or enjoy a hobby they've pursued all their lives.

Language problems. Everyone has trouble finding the right word now and then, but someone with Alzheimer's disease forgets simple words. For example, he or she may be unable to come up with the word *toothbrush* and instead will ask for "you know, that thing for my mouth."

Disorientation to time and place. We all occasionally forget what day of the week it is (especially if we don't read the newspaper) or that we were planning to go somewhere or do something on a particular date. But someone with Alzheimer's becomes lost on his or her own street, forgets where he is and how he got there, and has no idea how to get home.

Poor or impaired judgment. No one, not even my wife, always has perfect judgment. But those with Alzheimer's may dress inappropriately, wearing several shirts or blouses on a warm day, shorts in the wintertime, or a brown sock on one foot and a black one on the other. They often display poor judgment about money, giving away more than they can afford or buying products they don't really need or want.

Problems with abstract thinking. We all occasionally have trouble balancing a checkbook because of entry mistakes we've made or errors by the bank. Someone with Alzheimer's, however, forgets completely what the numbers are, what they mean, and what to do with them.

Misplacing things. It's common and normal to misplace a wallet or a set of keys, but a normal individual would never put an iron in the freezer or a wristwatch in the sugar bowl.

Changes in mood or behavior. It's normal to be sad or moody from time to time. Someone with Alzheimer's, on the other hand, has rapid mood swings—from happiness or calm to tears to anger—for no reason that's apparent to them or anyone else.

Changes in personality. While all of us change to some extent over the years, persons with Alzheimer's usually do so very obviously, becoming not only confused but also suspicious, fearful, paranoid, and progressively less independent.

Loss of initiative. It's normal to tire of your housework, business activities, or social obligations from time to time. That's usually a sign that you need a break or vacation. Someone with Alzheimer's, however, becomes very passive and withdrawn, spending his or her time just watching television or sleeping, without any interest or desire to perform any of his or her usual activities.

When these symptoms are full-blown, they're easy to recognize. However, it is key to recognize them. If you do recognize any of these warning signs—in a loved one or yourself—tell your doctor about it. Combined with the right computer software, a PET scan can reveal areas damaged by the tangles and build up of amyloid plaques that are the hallmarks of Alzheimer's. The cost of these diagnostic scans will be covered if they are needed to make a specific diagnosis. PET scans will be covered under U.S. government insurance (Medicare and Medicaid).

There is no way to stop Alzheimer's disease. It has been suggested that certain drugs such as Cognex (tacrine), Aricept (donepezil), Exelon (rivastigmine tartrate), Reminyl (galantamine)—either alone or in combination with the newest medication, Namenda (memantine)—might slow the progress of the disease in its early stages.

Frankly, I have not been impressed with their results in my own practice. But like most doctors, I prescribe them out of sheer desperation because there is little else that I can do for unfortunate individuals with AD.

Now comes a British study published in the journal *Lancet*, reporting that Aricept, the most commonly used of these drugs, does not, in fact, slow the progression of AD or affect the point at which patients must be admitted to nursing homes. These researchers claim that the studies funded by the manufacturers of these drugs suggesting otherwise are flawed. Although patients who took Aricpet did improve their performance on tests of mental and functional ability ("spell 'world' backward"), these improvements were of little significance. A more recent report from the Mayo Clinic, however, is somewhat more positive about Aricept. According to these researchers, Aricept given to patients with mild memory impairment (a forerunner of Alzheimer's), did delay the onset of frank AD by 18 months.

There are, however, medications that effectively control troublesome symptoms such as insomnia, agitation, wandering, anxiety, and depression. Although none of them slow the progress of Alzheimer's, they may make patients more comfortable and easier to care for.

There is some evidence that inflammation in the brain may contribute to the development of AD (see page 54). That's why some doctors prescribe nonsteroidal anti-inflammatory drugs (NSAIDs) to help prevent it in vulnerable individuals (those with the genes for AD or a strong family history). There is no evidence, however, that these agents are effective once symptoms of the disease have appeared.

THE BOTTOM LINE

Alzheimer's is a progressive neurological disorder of the elderly that is not part of the normal aging process. It is a disease in its own right. Although there is currently no cure for AD, several medications are available that can make life easier for those who suffer from Alzheimer's and for their caregivers by controlling burdensome symptoms. Early recognition is important so that preparations can be made for the most effective care once the disease is established.

The drugs now available to improve cognition and slow the progress of the disease have only a modest, time-limited effect, which is why most doctors continue to prescribe them (and patients' families ask for them). PET scans can help suggest the diagnosis and are now covered by Medicare and Medicaid. Remember, however, that there are several common disorders that mimic Alzheimer's. If you're given this diagnosis, make sure to get a second opinion from a good neurologist.

ARTHRITIS

· · · · · · · · · ·

Combination Treatment for Rheumatoid Arthritis

THE TERM *ARTHRITIS* is not a specific diagnosis. It simply means that one or more of your joints are inflamed, for which there are more than 100 different possible causes. For example, you may have been injured (traumatic arthritis), or you may have gout (gouty arthritis), or one of your joints may have been infected by any one of a number of agents, including gonorrhea. The two most common forms of arthritis, however, are osteoarthritis and rheumatoid arthritis.

Osteoarthritis is the result of long-standing wear and tear on the joints that develops usually as we grow older. It involves a loss of cartilage and a change in bone constitution. Rheumatoid arthritis is totally different and results from inflammation of the joints that have been attacked because of a faulty immune system. It affects more than 2.1 million Americans, of whom 1.5 million are women. It's progressive, chronic, and often crippling. It usually starts in middle age but may occur in children and young adults. Unlike osteoarthritis, which is confined to the joints, rheumatoid arthritis usually also involves internal organs such as the heart and lungs.

There are several ways to treat rheumatoid arthritis, but the first goal is to reduce symptoms—joint pain, stiffness, and swelling. This can be done with drugs such as aspirin, nonsteroidal anti-inflammatories (NSAIDs), and corticosteroids. Exercise, heat, cold, and physiotherapy also play an important role. In addition, a category of medications referred to as disease-modifying antirheumatic drugs (DMARDs) can affect the underlying disease process in addition to reducing pain. For the past 20 years, the DMARD of choice has been methotrexate (Rheumatrex), originally developed for the treatment of various cancers. Unfortunately, it is effective in only one in three patients with rheumatoid arthritis.

More recently, a new class of drugs—the prototype of which is Enbrel (etanercept)—has become available. It targets and neutralizes an inflammation-causing protein called tumor necrosis factor. Patients who don't respond to methotrexate are given Enbrel, but heretofore the drugs were not usually taken together.

Another form of therapy, called Prosorba, filters the blood of patients with rheumatoid arthritis and removes the inflammatory antibodies from the circulation. Older agents such as gold therapy, antimalarial medications, a variety of biologic agents, azathioprine (Azasan), and cyclosporine (Sandimmune) may also help. When joints have been badly damaged and are painful, and the patient is crippled and immobilized, surgery may be necessary.

HERE'S WHAT'S NEW

According to a report published in the *Lancet*, treating rheumatoid arthritis with a *combination* of methotrexate and Enbrel is more than twice as effective as either drug alone. Here are the data: After using both drugs for 1 year, 35 percent of 682 rheumatoid arthritis patients went into remission as compared with 13 percent of those on methotrexate alone and 16 percent taking only Enbrel. The other point to note is that all these patients had been suffering from the disease for years. It may be that starting this combination therapy sooner could slow down the rate of joint destruction and have an even greater effect.

THE BOTTOM LINE

There is no cure for rheumatoid arthritis. However, there are several different ways to reduce the joint pain, swelling, and deformity. Combining methotrexate and Enbrel, both of which affect the disease mechanism in addition to improving its symptoms, is more effective than either one alone. And the earlier this is done, the better.

The Latest Osteoarthritis Treatment

OSTEOARTHRITIS AFFECTS more than 20 million Americans and is a leading cause of disability in this country. An x-ray of the affected joint often indicates osteoarthritis even in the absence of any significant symptoms.

Osteoarthritis most commonly strikes the hips, knees, spine, and hands, and less frequently the elbows and shoulders. The onset of pain is usually gradual, and the joints are randomly involved—in contrast to rheumatoid arthritis, which affects both sides of the body. Both men and women can develop osteoarthritis of the hip, but women are more prone than men to have it in the knees and hands.

Unlike rheumatoid arthritis, osteoarthritis does not cause fever, weight loss, or anemia, or leave you feeling generally lousy. If you have any of these symptoms along with your joint pains, you probably have some other kind of arthritis.

How does osteoarthritis cause pain? Normally, the ends of the bones that meet to form the joint are covered by cartilage, a resilient, flexible tissue consisting mostly of water. Cartilage acts as a cushion between the bones, allowing them to move smoothly against each other. The bones and their cartilage are surrounded by a membrane filled with fluid (the *synovial* membrane), and the whole kit and caboodle is covered by a tough capsule that protects the entire joint from injury. Every time you move a normal joint, whether it's a finger or a hip, all these components interact with each other so that you can do so comfortably. But when you have osteoarthritis, the cartilage between the bones thins out, becomes stiff and rough, and loses its elasticity; the synovial membrane is irritated and makes too much fluid; and the bones form spurs. That's why an osteoarthritic joint is apt to be deformed, swollen, tender—and painful.

There are five key approaches to treating osteoarthritis.

Lose weight. Extra pounds put additional pressure on your joints.

Exercise. This strengthens the muscles that support the diseased joints. You should consult a good physiotherapist to prescribe the exercises that are right for you.

Apply heat and cold. Heat usually relaxes your muscles; cold relieves pain.

Medicate the pain. The mildest, over-the-counter drugs are used first—aspirin, acetaminophen, NSAIDs such as ibuprofen—and then stronger ones are prescribed as necessary. Remember that osteoarthritis is a chronic disease. Narcotics should be used only when absolutely necessary and, even then, sparingly in order to avoid dependence.

Topical ointments and creams can also ease pain; the most effective ones contain capsaicin derived from chile peppers. Glucosamine, with and without chondroitin, is also effective (see page 19), especially in women with osteoarthritis of the knees. Injection of hyaluronic acid into the knee can sometimes help, too. When joint pain is severe and does not respond to other drugs, corticosteroid injections into the joint are effective. This, however, should not be done more than three or four times a year. I have patients whose arthritic pain has been relieved by acupuncture as well as transcutaneous electrical nerve stimulation (TENS), which is administered by a small battery-powered unit that electrically stimulates local nerves, thus blocking pain signals to the spinal cord (and ultimately to the brain).

Consider surgery. This always should be a last resort. Techniques range from arthroscopic correction to joint replacement.

HERE'S WHAT'S NEW

Doctors at the Cardiff School of Biosciences at Cardiff University in Wales conducted an interesting study that suggests yet another approach to the treatment of osteoarthritis. They selected 31 patients with severe osteoarthritis of the knee who were awaiting knee replacement surgery. Half of them were given 1,000 milligrams of extra-strength cod liver oil daily, rich in omega-3 polyunsaturated fatty acids (the kind I recommend to protect the cardiovascular system). The other group received a placebo. Ten to 12 weeks after the surgery was performed, the researchers analyzed samples of cartilage and joint tissue taken from all the knees that had been replaced. They found that the knees from 86 percent of those who had taken the cod liver oil contained little or none of the enzymes that cause the cartilage damage and pain of osteoarthritis, as compared with 26 percent of those who had been taking a placebo capsule.

The Cardiff researchers consider these findings to be of major importance. They believe that these fish oils, which also prevent abnormal blood clotting, lower cholesterol, protect against sudden cardiac death, reduce the severity and frequency of asthmatic attacks, and lessen depression (see page 80), also slow down degeneration of the cartilage. In their opinion, adding omega-3 fish oils to your daily regimen will reduce pain and slow the progression of your osteoarthritis by virtue of their anti-inflammatory properties.

THE BOTTOM LINE

If you have osteoarthritis, eat lots of oily fish, such as salmon, fresh tuna, mackerel, kippers, sardines, and herring, or take omega-3 capsule supplements regularly. Their anti-inflammatory effects can slow down the progress of your osteoarthritis and help you in many other ways.

A Better Combination of Painkillers

OSTEOARTHRITIS IS THE MOST COMMON FORM of arthritis, affecting almost everyone after the age of 60. It is debilitating in some people but causes only minor aches and pains in others. Osteoarthritis is generally considered to be due to wear and tear of daily living. As discussed in the previous entry, treatment consists of painkillers, physiotherapy, appropriate use of heat and cold, and in some cases, joint replacement or other surgical measures.

When all's said and done, the most effective and safest nonnarcotic painkillers against osteoarthritis are the NSAIDs. The weaker strengths are available over the counter; stronger ones require a doctor's prescription. However, long-term use of NSAIDs, especially in the higher strengths, can irritate the intestinal tract and cause heartburn or bleeding, particularly in older people. So one always starts with the lowest effective dose.

Glucosamine, a popular nutritional supplement, also helps the pain of osteoarthritis, although not to the same extent as NSAIDs do. A sugar produced in the body and found in small amounts in foods (the shells of crabs, shrimps, and oysters), glucosamine plays an important role in maintaining healthy cartilage. As such, it's more than a painkiller; it helps prevent and repair damage to the bone and cartilage in the joint—and does so with minimal side effects. Many preparations of glucosamine contain chondroitin sulfate, which is said to boost its effectiveness.

The dosage of glucosamine is calculated on the basis of body weight. The recommended dose for most people is 500 milligrams three times a day. (If you weigh more than 200 pounds, you may need more. Discuss it with your doctor.) Take it with food to reduce the risk of upsetting your stomach. Also, glucosamine may interact with certain diuretics and require increasing their dose. If you're pregnant or breastfeeding, check with your doctor before taking glucosamine.

HERE'S WHAT'S NEW

According to a study at Temple University in Philadelphia, the results of which were published in the *Journal of Pharmacology and Experimental Therapeutics,* combining NSAIDs with glucosamine affords greater pain relief than when either medication is taken alone. Taking them together makes it possible to use lower doses of the NSAIDs with fewer side effects.

Here's how to do it. If you're already on a regular dose of an NSAID, add the glucosamine (either alone or along with chondroitin, although this particular study did not use the glucosamine-chondroitin combination). Since it takes a minimum of 2 weeks for the glucosamine to take effect, wait 2 to 3 weeks and then reduce the dose of the NSAID by half.

THE BOTTOM LINE

If you have been taking any NSAID (ibuprofen, naproxen, or one of the many others available) to relieve the pain of osteoarthritis, especially in strengths that require a prescription, try adding a 500-milligram glucosamine tablet three times a day. After 2 to 3 weeks, halve the dose of the NSAID. You may find that the lower dose may well control your pain.

CANCER

· · · · · · · · · · ·

A Drug That Starves Cancer

CANCERS REQUIRE A RICH BLOOD SUPPLY delivered through a network of blood vessels in order to continue their wild and deadly growth. Several years ago, a Harvard researcher named Judah Folkman, M.D., developed drugs that, when injected directly into a tumor, prevent these blood vessels from forming or expanding. His objective (and hope) was that by starving the malignancy, these agents would slow or prevent its spread.

In his experiments, Dr. Folkman was able to cure cancer-ridden mice with these anti-angiogenesis drugs (*angio* means "blood vessel"; *genesis* means "formation"). Unfortunately, he was unable to demonstrate any such effect in humans. The idea is so logical, however, that he and other researchers have continued the search for medications that can choke a tumor's blood supply. Clinical trials using several such agents have been in progress for years in patients with cancer of the lung, kidney, colon, and other organs.

HERE'S WHAT'S NEW

Dr. Folkman's idea works in humans! The FDA has approved one of these anti-angiogenesis drugs for the treatment of advanced colon cancer. The drug is called bevacizumab (where do they find these names?) and is mercifully marketed as Avastin. Two other agents, oxaliplatin (marketed as Eloxatin) and cetuximab (Erbitux), have also had an effect on these cancers, and clinical trials are in progress to determine how to combine them most effectively with existing chemotherapy regimens.

Here are the findings that prompted the FDA to approve Avastin: About 800 patients recently diagnosed with colorectal cancer and as yet untreated were divided into two groups. In the first, Avastin was added to standard anti-cancer chemotherapy. The others were given the same conventional medications but with a placebo instead of the Avastin. The median survival of patients on Avastin was about 20 months as compared with 15 months in those who received the placebo. Furthermore, the cancers in the Avastin-treated group were held in check for more than 10 months, while in the placebo recipients they spread within 6 months.

Avastin is not a cure, but this study is exciting because it shows that drugs that affect growth of blood vessels in a tumor *do* work. As we continue to learn how to use them, in what doses, and for which cancers, it is likely that these initial results will be replicated and possibly improve. In short, there's hope. A word of caution: Recent studies have also shown that Avastin may cause cardiovascular problems, so patients receiving this drug should have their cardiac status carefully monitored.

THE BOTTOM LINE

New treatments are being developed every day against cancer. The concept of attacking aggressive malignancies by cutting off their blood supply with drugs that prevent new vessels from forming within them (anti-angiogenesis) is an exciting one. Several different ones do so, and some have cured cancers in animals.

The approval of Avastin for the treatment of advanced colorectal cancer is a milestone because it is the first time that anti-angiogenesis has been shown to work, albeit temporarily, in humans. This holds promise of further progress. In the meantime, if you or someone you love has a colorectal malignancy too advanced to remove surgically, you may be able to buy some time. Discuss with your oncologist whether to add Avastin to your treatment regimen. Who knows? A more effective treatment may become available in the extra months of life that this agent can provide.

WHAT THE DOCTOR ORDERED?

FULL-BODY CAT SCANS: HOW SAFE ARE THEY?

I can't resist telling you this joke. Please forgive me. One day, a man who loved his dog very much found him lying motionless on the floor. Panic stricken, he rushed him to the vet. "What's wrong with my dog? He isn't moving."

The vet took one look at the dog and announced, "I'm sorry to tell you, but he's dead."

"That's impossible. We were playing together only last night. Are you sure?"

The vet left the room briefly, returned carrying a cat in his arms, and placed it beside the dog. The cat sniffed the dog's body for a few moments and then jumped off the table.

"That confirms it," said the vet. "Your dog is dead."

As he left the vet's office, the distraught man was presented with a bill for $500. "Five hundred dollars for a brief office visit? There must be some mistake!"

"Not at all," replied the vet. "That's what we charge for a CAT scan."

Computerized axial tomography (CAT) scanning, also called computed tomography (CT) scanning, is a diagnostic procedure that uses special x-ray equipment to obtain more-revealing pictures of various body organs such as the bowel, lungs, and heart. It is extremely useful in diagnosing and treating cancer. It enables the doctor to detect or confirm the presence of a tumor, as well as its size, its location, and information concerning whether it has spread. It can guide a biopsy and help plan radiation therapy or surgery, and it can help determine whether the cancer is responding to treatment.

A contrast agent or dye is often given before the CAT scan is done. It may be taken orally, injected into a vein, administered by an enema, or given in all three ways. Every now and then these contrast agents cause allergic reactions. Depending on the size of the area being x-rayed, the procedure may take from 15 minutes to 1 hour to complete. At the present time, most doctors recommend a CAT scan when a patient's history, symptoms, or physical findings suggest some type of abnormality, usually a tumor that requires further evaluation.

However, an increasing number of radiologists, most of whom have a financial interest in a medical imaging facility, are promoting another use for CAT scanning. They are urging healthy people *without any symptoms* to have their entire bodies scanned to detect (rather than to confirm) the presence of a tumor. The cost of such screening ranges from $500 to $1,200. These scans survey the body from the pelvis to the neck. (Head scans are usually done separately.)

The proponents of whole-body scans run advertisements containing testimonials from patients who describe how their disease was found early and that the scans saved their lives. These data are rejected as anecdotal because they lack scientifically rigorous studies.

The FDA has never approved, cleared, or certified any CAT system for such screening because it has never been demonstrated to save lives. Numerous professional organizations, including the American Heart Association, the American College of Cardiology, the American College of Radiology, and medical physicists at the American Association of Physicists in Medicine, are of the opinion that total-body scanning is "not scientifically justified" for patients *without* symptoms. They point out that in addition to the high cost of these procedures, which are not usually covered by insurance, these x-rays often result in false positive readings that can lead to needless surgery and cause potential complications.

Almost as an afterthought, they also point out that total-body scanning is associated with a "relatively high" level of radiation exposure. The magnitude of this exposure has never really been clarified. While a standard chest x-ray takes a single snapshot of the thorax, a CAT scanner takes multiple such views. The full-body scan also takes pictures along the length of the body rather than in just one targeted region. All this means a greater dose of ionizing radiation.

HERE'S WHAT'S NEW • The FDA reports (hold on to your seats for this one) that the radiation dose from *one* abdominal CT scan is equivalent to that from 100 to 150 chest x-rays! Imagine what the dose is from a total-body scan! An earlier study, admittedly controversial, attributed 2,500 deaths annually to excessive exposure to radiation from CT examinations.

Doctors at Yale University interviewed patients, emergency department physicians, and radiologists to determine whether they were aware of the radiation dose and possible risks associated with CAT scans. (In my own experience, few patients or even radiologists really give the amount of radiation exposure involved a second thought.) Only 7 percent of patients said that they had been told of the risks and benefits before their CAT scans, and only 22 percent of physicians admitted informing their patients of them. Only half of the *radiologists*—the experts doing these scans—are aware that they raise the lifetime risk of cancer, while 92 percent of patients (whom you can't really blame for not knowing) estimated the radiation dose of one CAT scan to be no more than that of 10 chest x-rays, as did 51 percent of the emergency room physicians and 61 percent of radiologists.

THE BOTTOM LINE • The CAT scan represents a major advance in diagnostic medicine. When it is used to clarify a potentially threatening symptom or finding that may require intervention, it is without parallel. However, its capricious use in healthy individuals does not justify the enormous amount of radiation exposure involved. My advice is to have a CAT scan of a specific organ when your doctor believes you need it. But don't have the screening body scan. It's not worth it.

Testicular Cancer Drug

WE HEAR SO MUCH ABOUT THE IMPORTANCE of early detection of breast cancer in women. Men get the short shrift as far as looking out for hormonal cancers is concerned, even though testicular cancer is diagnosed in an estimated 7,600 men each year. Men with an undescended testicle, abnormal testicular development, or those who've previously had cancer of the testicle are especially vulnerable to this malignancy.

As is true for any cancer, the successful treatment of testicular cancer depends on finding it before it has spread. The irony is that it is most common between 15 and 35 years of age, long before most men need to see a urologist for routine prostate checks. (These cancers can also occur in infancy and after 60 years of age, but that happens much less frequently.) The best way to find a testicular cancer is to look yourself for a painless, hard lump or enlargement of the testicle.

Treatment for testicular cancer involves removing the entire testicle and the cord that carries the sperm from it. Surgery is usually followed by radiation and chemotherapy. Testicular cancer can be cured even after it has spread to other parts of the body. However, there is some concern that the radiation therapy may predispose a person to the formation of other malignancies in the next 20 years, so anyone so treated should be carefully evaluated during that time.

HERE'S WHAT'S NEW

Researchers may have found an acceptable alternative to the radiation usually given after testicular cancer surgery. They studied some 1,400 patients with early such cancer, 900 of whom were treated with conventional radiation after their surgery; the remaining 500 received a single dose of the ovarian cancer drug carboplatin (Paraplatin) but no radiation. Three years later, there was only one man with a recurrence in the carboplatin-treated group, and seven in those who received radiation. (Carboplatin works by interfering with the growth of the cancer cells.)

THE BOTTOM LINE

If you have a testicular tumor and have been advised to have postoperative radiation, ask your doctor about taking one dose of carboplatin instead. The long-term results appear to be as good, but it doesn't have the future possible complications associated with radiation.

Detect Ovarian Cancer Early

OVARIAN CANCER is the fourth leading cause of cancer deaths among women in this country, killing 16,000 of them every year. Only lung, breast, and colorectal malignancies are more common. The irony is that 95 percent of women diagnosed with early-stage ovarian cancer survive at least 5 years. That's tantamount to a cure.

Ovarian cancer is so difficult to detect because the available ways to diagnose it, such as transvaginal ultrasound, are not really reliable. The blood test for CA-125, a marker for ovarian cancer, results in many false positives and false negatives. In other words, the test may be positive in the absence of ovarian cancer and fail to diagnose it when it is present. All these difficulties are compounded by the fact that this malignancy rarely causes telltale symptoms in time. The only sure way to diagnose the disease is to biopsy the ovary, and that's not a realistic option unless the suspicion of it being cancerous is very high. For all these reasons, 71 percent of ovarian cancers remain un-diagnosed until the disease has progressed to a point at which it is too late to cure.

HERE'S WHAT'S NEW

Over a 6-month period, doctors in Seattle analyzed a list of 20 symptoms reported by 1,709 cancer-free women whose average age was 45 years. They compared the symptoms these women reported during routine visits to their ob-gyn clinics with those reported by women who had ovarian cancer. They found three specific symptoms to be good indicators of ovarian cancer early in the disease as well as in advanced cases: (1) swollen abdomen, (2) a bloated feeling, and (3) an urgent need to urinate. These symptoms were present in 43 percent of women with ovarian cancer, but in only 8 percent who were cancer-free.

THE BOTTOM LINE

The sudden appearance, and persistence or worsening, of a swollen abdomen, abdominal bloating, and the need to urinate urgently for which no other cause is found should make you (and your doctor) consider the possibility of ovarian cancer, especially if you have a family history of this malignancy or breast cancer. Have a careful pelvic exam, then a transvaginal ultrasound and a CA-125 blood test. If these are all normal and the symptoms persist, discuss with your doctor whether to have a surgical look-see. The dire consequences of undiagnosed and untreated ovarian cancer justify an aggressive approach to its detection.

Prevent Melanoma with the Right Sunscreen

EVERYONE KNOWS THAT too much sun is harmful, that it can age the skin and cause everything from wrinkles to skin cancer. Unfortunately, that knowledge does not deter millions of us from the delicious experience of basking in the sun and getting a glorious tan that makes us the envy of all our cancer-free friends. We reassure ourselves that the sunscreens we apply in globs throughout the day will prevent damage to our skin.

HERE'S WHAT'S NEW

Confirming earlier observations by doctors at Memorial Sloan-Kettering Cancer Center in New York City, scientists in Great Britain have once more shown (and emphasized) that although sunscreens currently available in the United States do protect against the sun's ultraviolet B (UVB) rays, which cause skin malignancies such as basal cell carcinomas and squamous cell carcinomas, they do not offer adequate protection against its ultraviolet A (UVA) rays. These rays trigger the release of free radicals on the skin that ultimately lead to malignant melanoma, the most deadly form of skin cancer. (The incidence of malignant melanoma has been increasing 3 percent every year since 1981.)

These scientists worry that using the sunscreens available to us in the United States, even those with a high sun protection factor (SPF), may lull us into a sense of false security so that we take a much greater dose of the sun than is safe.

However, the experts at the American Academy of Dermatology are concerned that when sun worshippers learn that their sunscreens do not adequately protect them against UVA rays and malignant melanoma, they will use them less. They emphasize that these creams are important protection against all the skin problems caused by the sun, and that they should be continued along with the other measures such as avoiding excessive exposure to the sun and wearing protective clothing.

But a better answer may be on the way. Believe it or not, for several years the rest of the world—Europe, Asia, South America, Canada, Mexico, and Australia—has had access to a sunscreen that does protect against the dangerous UVA waves. The ingredient that does the trick is called Mexoryl (patented by the cosmetic maker L'Oréal). According to a senior dermatologist at New York University and past president of the American Academy of Dermatology,

Mexoryl is more than twice as effective as anything currently available here in the United States. I'm puzzled as to why it is not sold in this country and hope that the FDA will look into the matter, if it has not already done so. Until it does, you may be able to find Mexoryl at some pharmacies that sell imported sunscreens containing it.

THE BOTTOM LINE

The American Academy of Dermatology continues to emphasize the importance of liberally applying sunscreen with a high SPF when you're out in the sun, but warns that these lotions, creams, and ointments are but one tool to reduce damage to your skin and the risk of cancer. Also, they warn that sunscreens currently available in the United States do not adequately protect against malignant melanoma, the most dangerous kind of skin cancer, which is caused by UVA light. The sunscreen that does block these rays has been available in most of the rest of the world, including Canada. Its key ingredient is Mexoryl. Their main advice is to moderate your exposure to sunlight, continue to use whatever high SPF sunscreens are available, and wear protective clothing.

WHAT THE DOCTOR ORDERED?

ASPIRIN AND PANCREATIC CANCER • Aspirin is truly a wonder drug. It relieves pain and lowers fever. Its anticlotting properties help prevent strokes and heart attacks. It may delay the onset of Alzheimer's, and more recently it has been reported to reduce the incidence of various cancers—of the mouth, throat, esophagus (food pipe), lungs, prostate, colon, breast, ovary, and pancreas. (Its anticancer properties are believed to be due to the blocking of an enzyme called cyclooxygenase-2, which promotes inflammation and cancer growth.) Most doctors believe that we all should be taking aspirin regularly not only for prevention of vascular disease but also for its anti-cancer properties. That's why more than 20 million Americans use aspirin regularly.

HERE'S WHAT'S NEW • Recent studies have emphasized that aspirin's benefits, assumed to apply to everyone, may not work in from 5 percent to more than 40 percent of users in whom the aspirin does not stop the blood from clotting as it is supposed to do. The reasons for such resistance or nonresponsiveness are not fully understood and may be due to genetic or other factors. You can be tested to determine whether or not you are aspirin-resistant, but doctors do not agree whether people should do so or what to do about the results. This entire question is in limbo, but it has been raised, so you should be aware of it. When doctors have evidence of such aspirin resistance (for example, someone who has been taking it regularly nevertheless has another heart attack or stroke), they often prescribe another anticlotting medication called Plavix (clopidogrel). As great as aspirin is, there are alternatives.

Here's more news that's confusing doctors and their patients. On August 7, 2002, the *Journal of the National Cancer Institute,* a prestigious and respected publication, reported a study by researchers at the University of Minnesota in Minneapolis who evaluated some 28,000 postmenopausal women at regular intervals between 1992 and 1999. They focused on the use of aspirin during that period. The researchers found that women who took aspirin regularly had a 43 percent *lower* risk of pancreatic cancer than did those who did not use it at all.

Just as millions of women, braced by this news, started reaching for their aspirin bottles, researchers at the Roswell Park Cancer Institute in Buffalo, New York, completed a study in which they found that aspirin had *no effect* on the incidence of pancreatic cancer.

Now comes the coup de grâce. Harvard researchers, analyzing data from the Nurses' Health Study (which has provided invaluable information about a host of diseases in women over the years), concluded that taking aspirin regularly for years actually *increases* the risk of pancreatic cancer. This was no small fly-by-night research project. The Harvard scientists evaluated data collected over an 18-year period from 88,000 nurses and found that 161 of them developed pancreatic cancer. When they compared the characteristics of the afflicted women with those who remained cancer-free, they found that the greater the aspirin load (how many taken and for how long), the greater the risk of developing pancreatic cancer. For example, women who used only two or more aspirin a week but did so for 20 years or more had an 86 percent greater risk of pancreatic cancer than nonusers. On the other hand, one to three aspirin a week for a year or two conferred only an 11 percent greater risk.

So one study says there's no correlation between aspirin consumption and cancer of the pancreas, another says that aspirin reduces the risk, and a third says it is associated with a greater risk! Given this conflicting evidence, what's a doctor to tell a woman about aspirin—and what's a woman to do?

Remember that the conditions shown to benefit from aspirin are very much more common than is pancreatic cancer. French researchers recently reported that people who take aspirin for a heart condition have a high risk of serious cardiac problems when they discontinue it, even if they do so at their doctors' direction as before a tooth extraction, for example, or some type of surgery. In one large group who had been taking aspirin for a heart condition, 10 percent were hospitalized for heart attacks and other cardiac problems within a week after they discontinued it. The incidence of breast cancer is significantly reduced with regular use of aspirin (some say by as much as 50 percent), and this cancer is much more common than pancreatic cancer, which accounts for only 2 percent of all newly diagnosed cancers each year and no more than 5 percent of cancer deaths annually.

THE BOTTOM LINE • Despite the observation that some people may be resistant to aspirin, I am *not* advising my patients to change the way they currently use it. With regard to aspirin's role in the development of pancreatic cancer, there is no reason to believe that any of these conclusions—whether for or against aspirin—are wrong. Ongoing research will, in time, clarify the significance of these contradictory findings.

If you're taking aspirin because you have heart trouble, remember that heart disease is by far the biggest killer of men and women in this country. You're at many more times the risk of having a cardiac problem than you are of developing pancreatic cancer. If you're currently taking aspirin for any valid medical reason (and there are many), do not stop it for fear of developing pancreatic cancer. There are other safer ways to lessen your chances of developing this malignancy, notably, quitting tobacco and cutting down on your alcohol intake, both proven risk factors for this disease.

More Risk Factors for Breast Cancer

THERE ARE 1 MILLION NEW CASES of breast cancer every year worldwide, making it the most common malignancy in women (aside from skin cancer). It is the second leading cause of cancer mortality in the United States among females, with almost 200,000 new cases and some 40,000 deaths annually. (Lung cancer remains the number one cause of cancer deaths in American women.)

Women themselves can modify or eliminate some of the risk factors for breast cancer, such as hormone replacement therapy, alcohol consumption, and a fatty diet. Unfortunately, other important ones such as genetic makeup and family history are beyond their control. Having one or more risk factors does not necessarily mean that you will develop breast cancer. In fact, most women who are stricken with it are essentially risk-free. However, these risk factors do leave you more vulnerable, so it's important to control them whenever possible.

Following are the most important known risk factors for breast cancer.

Gender. Breast cancer is basically a woman's disease, although it also occurs in men (in far fewer numbers), especially those who are very overweight.

Age. The risk increases as you get older (18 percent of cases are in women in their forties; 77 percent occur in those 50 years or older).

Genes. Every woman has BRCA1 and BRCA2 genes whose function it is to *prevent* breast cancer. However, when these genes are altered (mutate), they increase a woman's risk of developing that malignancy. Such mutations are detectable with blood tests. These mutations give you a 35 to 85 percent chance of developing breast cancer (and ovarian cancer as well). Yet only 10 percent of women with breast cancer have these genes. Several other less common genes also predispose to breast cancer.

Family history. You're at greater risk if one or more blood relatives have or had breast or ovarian cancer, and especially if you are of Ashkenazi (Eastern Europe) Jewish heritage.

Previous breast cancer. If you've already had one bout of breast cancer, your risk of having a second one either in the same or the opposite breast is three to four times greater.

Race. Caucasian women are at slightly higher risk than African

Americans. On the other hand, Asian, Hispanic, and Native American females are less vulnerable.

Previous radiation. If you received any radiation treatment as a child or young adult for another cancer such as Hodgkin's disease or non-Hodgkin's lymphoma, you may be as much as 12 times more likely to develop breast cancer.

Menstrual periods. If your periods started before age 12 or ended after age 55, your risk is slightly greater. (That's presumably because of greater exposure to estrogen during your lifetime.)

Oral contraceptives. Whether or not they are associated with an increased cancer risk is still up in the air. But if you are at greater risk because of other risk factors, I suggest you choose another method of birth control.

No children. If you are childless or had your first baby after the age of 30, you're at slightly higher risk.

Hormone replacement therapy. Taking combined estrogen and progesterone for several years after menopause increases the risk of death from breast cancer. That risk virtually disappears 5 years after you stop taking these hormones.

Breastfeeding. The risk of having breast cancer is reduced if you breastfeed for at least 18 months to 2 years. (That's because, like pregnancy, nursing lowers the duration of exposure to estrogen associated with fewer menstrual cycles.)

Alcohol. The more alcohol you drink, the greater the risk of breast cancer.

Obesity. If you've gained weight as an adult, your breast cancer risk is greater, especially after age 50. (That's probably because overweight women have higher levels of estrogen.)

Dietary fat. Whether a fatty diet leads to breast cancer is still being debated. Most studies suggest that it does. Until the final evidence is in, my advice is to limit your fat intake. Better safe than sorry.

Exercise. Research is ongoing here, too, but regular moderate-to-strenuous exercise started early and continued into adult life probably protects against breast cancer.

Smoking. Tobacco may increase the risk for women who started smoking early in life, but there is no hard evidence that it does so. (However, there are enough other reasons to quit.)

The best chance of surviving breast cancer is to detect it as early as possible. That's why every female, regardless of her particular vulnerability, should have an annual mammogram (and, when needed, a breast sonogram or MRI as well) starting at age 40 and continuing for as long as her life expectancy is at least 10 years.

Younger women at increased risk should have mammography before age 40 years. Those with BRCA1 or BRCA2 mutations should begin having mammograms at age 25, or 10 years earlier than the youngest age at which breast cancer has been diagnosed in other members of their immediate family.

In addition to these tests, make sure your doctor also exams your breast manually. Ten percent of breast cancers are detected by such an examination even when the mammogram is "normal." An MRI is even more sensitive than a mammogram but considered too expensive to use for routine screening purposes.

HERE'S WHAT'S NEW

As if the list of risk factors listed above wasn't long enough, two more have recently been determined to increase your chances of developing breast cancer.

In the Harvard Nurses' Health Study of more than 116,000 women followed for many years, 6,000 had type 2 diabetes. Those among them who were menopausal had a 17 percent higher incidence of breast cancer than women whose blood sugar was normal. Researchers believe that higher blood-insulin levels in women with type 2 diabetes contribute in some way to the risk of the malignancy.

In a 1999 study of 10,000 women, Finnish scientists observed a higher incidence of breast cancer among those who frequently used antibiotics. Now, scientists at the University of Washington in Seattle have come up with a similar observation. The greater the frequency and number of antibiotics consumed, the higher the risk. This association was true for every kind of antibiotic, including penicillin, for whatever reason it was used—ranging from acne to respiratory infections. This is a significant finding. Hormone replacement therapy, whose dangers we hear so much about, is statistically less important a risk than is antibiotic use.

The key unanswered question is whether this association between antibiotics and breast cancer is due to the antibiotics themselves or the infections for which they were being taken. It is possible that women who never need antibiotics are "healthier" and have better immune systems than those who need them frequently. I'd like to see a similar study in men looking for some correlation between antibiotics and, say, prostate cancer.

THE BOTTOM LINE

I have listed 17 previously documented risk factors for breast cancer and added 2 new ones. Even though most cases of this malignancy occur in women without any risk factors, it pays to eliminate any that you happen to have. The latest additions—type 2 diabetes and antibiotics—are to some extent manageable. Diet and weight loss reduce the chances of developing type 2 diabetes, and so may lower your breast cancer risk.

As far as antibiotic use is concerned, it's not yet clear why it is associated with a greater likelihood of breast cancer. It may be the drugs themselves, the infections they're treating, or the fact that women who don't take antibiotics are more resistant to disease generally, including cancer. So take an antibiotic if you need it, but don't let it become a crutch for mild infections, such as the common cold, cough, or other viral infections that do not respond to them. Remember, antibiotics are not the harmless chicken soup your grandmother fed you whenever you caught cold.

When Breast Cancer Is in Your Genes

THERE ARE MANY RISK FACTORS for breast cancer (see page 34), key among which are your family history and genetics. If your mother, sisters, or other close blood relatives had breast cancer, you are more likely to be stricken, too. This risk can be further established by testing for the presence of the mutated BRCA1 and BRCA2 genes (BRCA is the abbreviation for breast cancer).

These genes are normally present in healthy women, and they *prevent* tumor formation by helping repair damaged DNA. However, women in whom these genes have mutated (changed their normal structure) are at much higher risk for developing breast cancer than are women without these mutations. (Fortunately, only 10 percent of women with breast cancer carry these mutated genes.) By the time a woman with a mutated BRCA1 or BRCA2 gene reaches the age of 80, she will have had an 82 percent chance of developing breast cancer. Women with the BRCA1 mutation also have a 54 percent risk of ovarian cancer, while those harboring the BRCA2 mutation have a 23 percent risk. (Only 2 percent of women free of this mutation are at risk for this malignancy.)

What should you do if you have the mutated BRCA1 or BRCA2 gene? Are having more frequent screenings for breast cancer and changing your lifestyle to eliminate other risk factors enough to protect you?

HERE'S WHAT'S NEW

Every woman should have a yearly mammogram after age 40, and earlier than that if she has any special risk factors. If, however, you carry the mutation of the BRCA1 or BRCA2 gene (it's especially common among Ashkenazi Jewish women), you should have a mammogram sooner and more often. In a recent study at Columbia-Presbyterian Hospital in New York City, almost half of these mutated-gene carriers developed evidence of breast cancer an average of 5 months after their last normal annual mammogram, during which time the cancer had sometimes already spread to the lymph nodes. So doctors are now recommending that such women have a mammogram at least every 6 months, and preferably every 4.

There were some interesting results published in the *Journal of Clinical Oncology* from an international study of the long-term follow-up of 483 women with these BRCA mutations, some of whom had undergone "preventive" mastectomy of both breasts, and others had not. Six years later, only 2 of the 105 women (1.9 percent) who had undergone the surgery developed breast cancer. By contrast, 184 of the 378 women who had opted for watchful waiting developed it. Similar results were obtained in other studies.

It would appear that the most effective way to protect yourself against breast cancer if you have the BRCA1 or BRCA2 gene mutation is to have both breasts removed (bilateral mastectomy). This is a difficult and painful decision to make. Women who reject so drastic an approach can instead take prophylactic tamoxifen (Nolvadex) for 5 years, all the while being closely monitored by mammography or other imaging tests. This drug may reduce the chances of breast cancer by half in high-risk women. Tamoxifen, however, is not without side effects (see page 42).

There are other options besides bilateral mastectomy. According to a recent study published in *Plastic and Reconstructive Surgery*, the official medical journal of the American Society of Plastic Surgeons, *breast-reduction* surgery may be a desirable alternative. Enough breast tissue is removed to substantially lower the risk of developing breast cancer, although not to the same extent as does the more extensive operation. A recent analysis of results in 32,000 women who underwent such breast reduction revealed a 50 to 70 percent lower incidence of subsequent breast cancer. Also, because some breast tissue is preserved, the results are more cosmetically acceptable to many women than those obtained after total bilateral mastectomy. Although the protection is not as great with this compromise, it's substantially better than no intervention at all.

There is yet another option for such women. New research from the Center for Research in Women's Health in Toronto published in the *Journal of the National Cancer Institute* reveals that women with the mutated BRCA1 gene who breastfeed their children for more than 1 year are about 60 percent less likely to develop breast cancer than those who don't. Although that's significant protection, their risk still remains high. The reason for this benefit no doubt relates to the level of estrogen exposure. The less time estrogen levels are high, the lower their risk. (Estrogen levels fall during pregnancy and stay low during breastfeeding.)

If you have bad breast genes, you may also want to consider removal of your ovaries after you're done having children. Cancer of the ovary, unlike that of the breast, is very difficult to detect, and there is currently no reliable screening test to detect it. Ninety percent of patients with this malignancy die within 5 years after the diagnosis is made, even though it can be cured if caught in time. Unfortunately, it rarely is. Removal of the ovaries will leave you in a menopausal state, but that's a small price to pay for survival.

THE BOTTOM LINE

If you carry the mutated BRCA1 or BRCA2 gene, you should have a mammogram at least every 6 months, and preferably every 4.

Abnormal BRCA genes are responsible for only 10 percent of all breast (and many ovarian) cancers, but the chances of developing such a malignancy is very great if you have them. Removing both breasts reduces the chance of breast cancer by more than 90 percent. Less extensive breast-reduction surgery yields more satisfactory cosmetic results but offers only a 50 to 70 percent lower risk. If you're having children, you should breastfeed them as long as possible. Consider all these measures carefully. And while you're at it, also weigh the pros and cons of having your ovaries removed after you've finished having your family, in order to forestall getting this deadly cancer, too.

A Better Breast-Cancer Treatment

IN TWO-THIRDS of postmenopausal women with breast cancer, the malignant cells are stimulated by estrogen. Tamoxifen (Nolvadex), an estrogen-blocking drug, cuts the recurrence rate of the cancer by half after the cancer has been surgically removed. But there are problems with this drug, the main one being that it is no longer protective after 5 years. It also increases the risk of blood clotting in women confined to bed for long periods, especially after surgery, and it predisposes to cancer of the uterus. Despite these and other side effects, the overall benefits of tamoxifen in controlling serious complications of breast cancer far outweigh its drawbacks.

HERE'S WHAT'S NEW

Three new anti-estrogen drugs—called aromatase inhibitors and marketed as Aromasin (exemestane), Femara (letrozole), and Arimidex (anastrozole)—protect cancer patients even more than tamoxifen does and with fewer adverse effects. They work by inhibiting a natural enzyme in the body called aromatase, which helps make estrogen. By blocking this enzyme, these drugs reduce the amount of estrogen available to stimulate the breast cancer cells.

In a large international study of almost 5,000 postmenopausal women with breast cancer, which was reported in the *New England Journal of Medicine,* roughly half took tamoxifen for 2 to 3 years and were then switched to one of these aromatase inhibitors (Aromasin); the rest continued with tamoxifen. After 31 months, the women who took the Aromasin had 32 percent fewer recurrences or spread of their cancer than those who continued on tamoxifen alone. They also had half as many new cancers develop in the other breast than did the tamoxifen-only group.

Last year, in a smaller study of postmenopausal women with estrogen-sensitive breast cancer, all of whom had completed a 5-year course of tamoxifen, those who continued with Femara (another aromatase inhibitor) had 50 percent fewer recurrences of their cancer than patients who simply stopped the tamoxifen without any further therapy.

There is ongoing research on these aromatase inhibitors to see whether they can *prevent* breast cancer in women with a bad family history or genetic vulnerability to the disease. Their main adverse effect appears to be increased bone loss.

To give you some idea how quickly important new breakthroughs occur in medicine, no sooner had I finished writing the first draft of this piece than doctors at the Duke Comprehensive Cancer Center in Durham, North Carolina, presented new findings at the annual

American Society of Clinical Oncology meeting. They have been using a new and experimental breast cancer drug called lapatinib in women whose tumors did not respond to other traditional therapies, including Herceptin (trastuzumab, which is the frontline drug used to treat tumors that produce too much of the growth-regulating protein called Her2). Lapatinib is a new type of therapy that targets and blocks the action of *two* growth factors that stimulate breast cancer cells. According to this latest study, in 46 percent of breast cancer patients who took this (oral) drug for 8 weeks, the disease either remained stable or the tumor shrank, as it did in 24 percent of those who received it for 4 months.

Finally, another observation may have a bearing on interpreting the efficacy of tamoxifen. New research indicates that 40 percent of women have a genetic mutation that interferes with tamoxifen. Certain antidepressants may also do so. So any woman with breast cancer who is taking antidepressants along with tamoxifen should be observed for any waning of tamoxifen's effects. It has not yet been determined whether this interaction also exists with the aromatase inhibitors.

THE BOTTOM LINE

Tamoxifen, an anti-estrogen drug, continues to be very useful for the prevention, recurrence, or spread of breast cancer in postmenopausal women whose tumors are fueled by estrogen. However, a new and different class of estrogen blockers, called aromatase inhibitors, is also protective.

More research is needed to determine whether (1) tamoxifen should be abandoned and women should instead start taking an aromatase inhibitor immediately after breast cancer surgery, (2) they should take tamoxifen for 2 or 3 years and then switch, or (3) they should take tamoxifen for the full 5 years and then continue with the aromatase inhibitor. Oncologists are leaning toward the second option. But stay tuned; it is entirely possible that ongoing studies will conclude that these aromatase inhibitors should replace tamoxifen altogether. The possible adverse effects of antidepressants on tamoxifen should also be considered in women taking both types of medication.

In the meantime, if you are taking tamoxifen because of breast cancer, discuss with your doctor whether you should switch to an aromatase inhibitor. If you do so, look out for osteoporosis and take one of the many medications available to slow its progress or prevent it. Note that neither tamoxifen nor aromatase inhibitors should be used by *premenopausal* women or those whose breast cancers are not estrogen dependent.

A newer, still experimental drug called lapatinib was reported by doctors at Duke University to be effective in controlling two growth factors that stimulate breast cancer cells.

The larger message I want to impart is that effective new therapies are being developed all the time and that we will surely conquer breast cancer one day.

Breast Cancer Surgery—More May Not Be Better

UNTIL RELATIVELY RECENTLY, it was considered prudent and necessary for a woman with breast cancer to have her entire breast removed (mastectomy) rather than just the tumor itself. After all, if there was any question, why take the chance of leaving behind any tissue that might be harboring stray malignant cells? But with experience, it became clear that such megasurgery was overkill and that breast cancers could be cured by (1) removing a discrete malignancy and leaving the rest of the gland intact (lumpectomy), (2) checking for and removing lymph nodes in the arm, and then (3) undergoing a course of radiation. These three steps seemed to be enough, provided, of course, that the "margins" of the tumor were clean, and no lumps or other evidence of tumor remained elsewhere in the breast.

Today most women with early, localized breast cancer choose lumpectomy. However, some have lingering doubts as to whether they made the right decision. Would it have been safer to remove the breast and be done with it?

HERE'S WHAT'S NEW

If you've had a lumpectomy, you can stop worrying. Scientists at the National Cancer Institute recently reevaluated 237 women who had been operated on for early breast cancer during the past 20 years—58 percent of them had undergone mastectomies; 52 percent chose lumpectomy along with removal of lymph nodes and postoperative radiation. (Some women with lumpectomies later went on to have mastectomies when other tumors were detected in their breasts.)

The good news is that there was no difference in survival in the lumpectomy and mastectomy patients after 20 years.

The doctors emphasize the need for continued surveillance after lumpectomy because of the possibility of new malignancies developing in the remaining breast tissue. Even after a mastectomy, such follow-up examinations are also necessary to make sure a tumor has not appeared in the other breast. If, however, new lesions that are found after either procedure are dealt with promptly, the mastectomy does not appear to have any advantage over the simpler lumpectomy.

Here's another piece of news of which you should be aware. Researchers at the University of Pennsylvania in Philadelphia conducted a study at 17 different sites throughout the United States, Canada, and Germany in which they studied 1,000 women, most of whom were older than 40, for a period of 3 years. All these women had sus-

picious lesions on their mammograms that required further evaluation to see if they were cancerous. All of them were evaluated with
mammograms and magnetic resonance imaging (MRI). Cancer was
detected in 428 of these women. The MRI was found to be more
than twice as effective as mammography in finding multiple tumors.
(MRI is a noninvasive procedure that uses powerful magnets and
radio waves to construct pictures of the part of the body being
studied. It uses the magnetic properties of atoms to differentiate between possible benign and malignant tissue.)

So what are we to conclude? If you have breast cancer and are
trying to decide what kind of surgery to have, it's very important that
you have an MRI before making up your mind. The MRI is a must
in order to detect the full extent of the breast cancer before surgery
so that you can preserve as much healthy breast tissue as possible.
These findings will even further improve the effectiveness of lumpectomy by reducing the risk of missing other, smaller tumors.

Another recent report will make lumpectomy an even easier
choice. Typically, postoperative radiation is given externally 5 days a
week over a 6-week period. There is a new approach, called balloon
brachytherapy, that delivers the radiation to the area from which the
malignant tumor was removed and not to the entire breast. A small
balloon device, called the MammoSite catheter, is inserted through a
skin incision into the area from which the cancer was removed. The
balloon is then inflated and radioactive material inserted that radi-
ates the area twice a day for 5 days. After the treatment is completed,
the balloon is deflated and removed.

According to doctors at Rush University Medical Center in
Chicago, this limited breast radiation is as effective as radiating the
entire breast. The shortened treatment time is also more convenient.
During a 1- to 2-year follow-up of 112 women over age 40 treated

with balloon brachytherapy, there were no cancer recurrences. Long-term results are being accumulated.

THE BOTTOM LINE

Women with early, localized breast cancer have the same long-term cure rate from lumpectomy followed by lymph node removal and radiation as do those who undergo the modified mastectomy. Both groups, however, require ongoing surveillance. Before choosing lumpectomy, you should have an MRI of the breast. It is more sensitive than mammography to detect the presence of other cancers in the breast that should also be removed. A shorter method of postoperative radiation, 1 week of treatment rather than 6, described above should also be considered.

Treating Noninvasive Breast Cancer

THERE ARE SEVERAL DIFFERENT TYPES of breast cancer. Although some are more aggressive than others, they must all be removed surgically. The next step varies—some patients then do best with postoperative radiation; others, with chemotherapy, depending on the size of the cancer, its cell type, its location in the breast, its dependence on hormones (estrogen), whether or not it has already spread to glands in the armpit or elsewhere, the patient's genetics, and other factors. So before deciding what therapy is best for you, be sure to ask your doctor about the characteristics of your particular kind of breast cancer and what your treatment options are.

Currently, 25 to 30 percent of all reported breast cancers are the type referred to as ductal carcinoma in situ (DCIS), occurring in more than 55,000 women every year in the United States. DCIS involves the cells lining the ducts through which milk flows to the nipple. It is almost always detected by mammography, not by physical exam, because it remains so small for so long. In fact, before mammography became routine and so widespread, DCIS was thought to be uncommon and to represent only 3 percent of cancers. In those days, it was diagnosed only when a small lump or a nipple discharge was observed.

Mammography now detects these cancers by revealing the presence of microcalcifications before the tumor is large enough to feel. But if you are told that there are such microcalcifications in your mammogram, don't panic. Most of them are benign and do not reflect DCIS. Why such calcifications occur in a noncancerous breast is not always clear. It may be a sign of aging or due to the deposition of calcium in the small blood vessels within the breast tissue. But an experienced radiologist can usually tell from looking at them under magnification whether they are harmless or possibly indicate underlying DCIS. As a rule, the larger, smoother, and more rounded these microcalcifications are, the less likely they reflect malignant disease. However, it's the radiologist's call. If there is any doubt about their significance, you'll need a biopsy.

Every DCIS is "staged" in several different ways—"stage zero" is the earliest form, next is "precancerous," then "preinvasive," followed by "noninvasive" or "*intra*ductal" cancer. Although still localized, the higher the grade, the more likely it is to spread.

In addition to the *stage* of the tumor, there are three different recognizable *grades*—low, intermediate, and high. The higher the grade, the more likely DCIS is to become invasive. Although some of these cells are not destined to spread, we remove them all since we can't be sure which ones will and which won't spread. The good news is that only 2 percent of patients with DCIS who are treated die of breast cancer within 10 years.

DCIS is always treated surgically. Only the portion of the breast tissue that contains the tumor is removed, along with a margin of normal breast tissue around it, just to be sure the surgeon has gotten all of it. The rest of the breast is left intact. This operation is called a wide local excision. Although many doctors believe follow-up radiation is necessary, others don't. Who's right?

HERE'S WHAT'S NEW

Doctors at the Dana-Farber Cancer Institute and Brigham and Women's Hospital, both in Boston, have found that surgery alone to remove DCIS is *not* enough, even when these cancers are caught early and very small. They monitored 157 such patients who did not have radiation after surgery for an average of $3^{1}/_{2}$ years. Thirteen had recurrences of the original cancer in the same breast; 9 developed another DCIS in a different location within the breast; and in 4 patients, the cancer had spread outside the milk ducts into breast tissues. Although there was no control group with which to compare the results in this particular study, this recurrence incidence of almost 10 percent is higher than what is usually observed in patients who also receive radiation. The doctors doing this study were sufficiently impressed to recommend that surgery of DCIS be followed by radiation.

THE BOTTOM LINE

DCIS is usually a slow-growing form of breast cancer and does not always invade surrounding breast tissue. However, it must be removed because we cannot predict if and when it will spread. Doctors used to think that simply excising the tumor was enough to cure it. But when localized excision of the tumor is followed by postoperative radiation, the incidence of recurrence or spread appears to be significantly reduced. Be sure to discuss this option and the findings of the Boston researchers with your doctor.

WHAT THE DOCTOR ORDERED?

BLACK COHOSH, BY GOSH ● Until quite recently, women had no qualms about hormone replacement therapy (HRT) to relieve their menopausal symptoms, the most prominent and persistent of which are hot flashes. HRT also reduces the likelihood of osteoporosis. But then came the barrage of new findings warning that, while HRT does ease the unpleasant consequences of menopause, its downside may not be worth it. Statistically, over the long term the hormone supplements raise the risk of breast cancer, heart disease, and stroke. So doctors now prescribe HRT only when the side effects of menopause are unbearable, and then only at the lowest effective dose for the shortest period of time.

Now that HRT is no longer routinely recommended, menopausal women have been looking for an effective alternative. There is a plethora of products being touted for relief of menopausal symptoms, ranging from a variety of soy preparations to other synthetic estrogens. I am not aware that any have been shown to be effective.

Black cohosh, a member of the buttercup family and native to North America, is an herb sold as a dietary supplement. It was used by Native Americans, mainly as an insect repellent but also as a diuretic and for a variety of gynecological disorders, kidney problems, rheumatism, sore throat, and for bringing on delayed menstruation. (Readers of a certain age will be interested to know that black cohosh was the major ingredient—along with lots of alcohol—in Lydia E. Pinkham's Vegetable Compound that was so popular with women many years ago.)

In 2001, the American College of Obstetricians and Gynecologists concluded that black cohosh might be helpful over the short term (6 months or less). The German Federal Institute for Drugs and Medical Devices Commission E has approved it for treating menopausal symptoms and painful menstruation (which means that its cost is reimbursed by the German government). Countless thousands of menopausal women in this country are taking black cohosh.

The mode of action of black cohosh remains unknown, but it does contain many potentially biologically active substances. However—and this is important in view of what you will read below—one of them, fukinolic acid, has estrogenic activity. This raises the concern that long-term use of black cohosh may affect the uterus and breast. For this reason, a National Institutes of Health (NIH) committee currently conducting a study on the effectiveness of black cohosh for treating menopausal symptoms has advised pregnant women and those with breast cancer not to take it. I'm not sure how widely and aggressively that advice has been publicized, because as best I can tell (especially from visiting neighborhood health food stores), the herb is selling like hotcakes.

HERE'S WHAT'S NEW • The results of a study presented at the 94th annual meeting of the American Association for Cancer Research reported that breast tumors in mice who were fed black cohosh in a dosage comparable to the 40 milligrams per day that women take for menopausal symptoms were three times more likely to spread than those in mice not given black cohosh. This suggests the possibility that women with documented breast cancer should not be taking black cohosh.

According to the Center for Science in the Public Interest (CSPI), preliminary research suggests that black cohosh may increase the risk of liver failure and cause breast cancer to spread. It has suggested to the NIH that even those women participating in its ongoing study of black cohosh be warned about these dangers. (Labels on commercially sold bottles of black cohosh do caution pregnant women and nursing mothers not to take the herb but do not mention its possible effect on breast cancer or liver function.)

THE BOTTOM LINE • Until further studies are completed, I don't think it's a good idea for postmenopausal women to take black cohosh. Remember that much human research starts with animals, especially mice; some of the most important observations over the years were first made in mouse experiments. There is evidence that black cohosh, already suspected of having estrogenic properties (and estrogen is known to be a risk factor for breast cancer), spreads existing breast cancer in mice. That being the case, no woman with or without breast cancer should take black cohosh until current studies about its safety have been completed.

C-Reactive Protein and Colon Cancer

THE BLOOD LEVEL of C-reactive protein (C-RP), a protein made by the liver, has been used for many years as an indicator of inflammation anywhere in the body. However, its value in specifically predicting susceptibility to heart attacks has been only recently appreciated. In last year's edition of *Breakthrough Health,* I reported that men and women with elevated C-RP are more vulnerable to premature heart attacks, strokes, and diabetes. I recommended that C-RP testing be part of every routine cardiovascular evaluation and that elevated levels (3 or higher) should prompt a very aggressive prevention program to reduce the likelihood of a heart attack or stroke. Preventive measures include weight reduction, exercise, normalization of cholesterol and related values, smoking cessation, and treatment of high blood pressure.

Knowing the C-RP level is important because the inflammation it reflects is the response of living tissue to damage of any type—from physical injury, toxins, chemicals, or infections. Such inflammation, often silent, may be the forerunner of many different diseases, including Alzheimer's and cancer. Treating the inflammation with anti-inflammatory agents such as aspirin or nonsteroidal anti-inflammatory drugs (NSAIDs) such as ibuprofen may halt progression of whatever condition the inflammation reflects.

HERE'S WHAT'S NEW

C-RP may signal increased risk not only for heart disease but also for colon cancer. Blood samples from 500 adults obtained by researchers at the Johns Hopkins Medical Institutions in Baltimore between 1989 and the end of 2000 revealed that those with the highest C-RP levels were $2^1/_2$ times more likely to develop colon cancer than those with the lowest readings.

Researchers at Duke University have also found that otherwise healthy people who are prone to anger, hostility, and mild depression produce higher levels of C-RP. This could account for their increased risk for cardiovascular disease and stroke, even in the absence of other traditional risk factors. We have known for some time that depressed men and women suffer more cardiac events and early death.

THE BOTTOM LINE

If these observations are confirmed by further studies (as I expect they will be), the results of your routine C-RP testing should be considered when assessing your risk for not only vascular disease and diabetes but also colon cancer. If your reading is abnormally high, you and your doctor should discuss more frequent testing for colon cancer, utilizing examination of the stool for the presence of blood, colonoscopy (a procedure in which the entire colon is viewed), or sigmoidoscopy (one that examines the lower third of the colon). Ask about prophylactic maintenance therapy with one of the NSAIDs, especially if you have a family history of bowel cancer or previously had any polyps removed. You should also take a hard look at your behavior patterns and get the necessary help to "calm down and be happy."

Virtual Colonoscopy—Not Ready for Prime Time

SCREENING FOR COLON CANCER when appropriate—in vulnerable people, at the right time, at optimal intervals, and in the right age groups—can lead to early detection, treatment, and cure. There are currently four major screening techniques available for people over the age of 50.

- Fecal occult blood test: a routine annual examination of the stool to detect the presence of blood (not always visible to the naked eye)

- Sigmoidoscopy: a procedure performed every 5 years (except in people who subsequently develop symptoms later on, or in whom one or more polyps were found, or those who are especially vulnerable by virtue of a strong family history of colorectal cancer)

- Colonoscopy: a procedure done every 10 years (with the same exceptions as those for sigmoidoscopy)

- Virtual colonoscopy: a test not yet part of the screening regimen recommended by the American Cancer Society

Virtual colonoscopy is the most recent technique developed to examine the bowel. It is minimally invasive, and it does not require sedation. The patient is spared the discomfort of the 5-foot-long tube used during a conventional colonoscopy. Instead, the colon is filled with air through a small tube inserted into the anus. A CT scan then visualizes the large bowel after the introduction of air into the bowel. This procedure also avoids accidental perforation of the bowel, which occasionally complicates conventional colonoscopy.

I don't refer many patients for virtual colonoscopy. In my opinion, the worst part of any colonoscopy is the preparation—the laxatives and enemas to clean the bowel. This is required for both the conventional and the virtual procedures. Also, if the doctor finds a polyp during the conventional test, it can be removed right then and there. In the virtual procedure, the whole cleansing preparation must be repeated and the patient brought back for a conventional colonoscopy anyway.

HERE'S WHAT'S NEW

A study conducted at the Medical University of South Carolina in Charleston compared the results on 615 adults age 50 and older who underwent routine virtual colonoscopy at nine major hospitals. This procedure was then followed by conventional colonoscopy. When the patients were asked which of the techniques they preferred, 46 percent chose the CT procedure, and 41 percent chose the conventional colonoscopy. But this was more than a popularity contest. The researchers were interested in the *accuracy* of the two procedures. They found that virtual colonoscopy detected only 55 percent of growths that were at least 10 millimeters in size, and only 39 percent of smaller polyps at least 6 millimeters in diameter. By contrast, the accuracy of conventional colonoscopy was almost 100 percent. Also, two of eight cancers were missed by virtual colonoscopy.

This difference in the reliability of the two techniques is believed to be due to the current lack of experience among doctors performing virtual colonoscopies in this country. There is no assurance that, despite all their advertising, these physicians are sufficiently well trained. There is also a real question as to how long it will take before enough doctors achieve the degree of expertise necessary to interpret virtual colonoscopy results accurately.

THE BOTTOM LINE

Properly interpreted CT virtual colonoscopy is as accurate as the conventional technique. There are advantages and disadvantages to both as far as patients are concerned. In my own practice, I recommend conventional colonoscopy because it allows the doctor to remove then and there any polyps that are present. By contrast, if a growth is found during virtual colonoscopy, the patient has to come back and undergo the conventional technique in order to remove it. But more important than that, except for certain sophisticated specialized centers, the accuracy of the findings in virtual colonoscopy is suspect because of the lack of expertise by many doctors doing this test. If you're going to have your bowel examined, I recommend the conventional colonoscopy.

The Best Way to Cure Early Colon Cancer

THERE IS A GREAT DEAL OF INTEREST in how to prevent or reduce the chances of developing colon cancer, a major killer of men and women in this country. The best way to cure such a malignancy is to remove it surgically as soon as possible. Follow-up chemotherapy and radiation may be necessary if the tumor has spread.

Bowel cancer surgery has traditionally been an open operation. In other words, the abdomen is exposed and explored, and the offending growth is removed. This is major surgery that disturbs bowel function and requires patients to stay several days in the hospital. Is laparoscopic, or "keyhole," surgery—now so widely used to remove gallbladders, appendixes, and a host of growths—a feasible alternative for colon cancer? Laparoscopy is much less complicated, recovery from it is faster, and patients can leave the hospital much sooner. It requires only a few very small incisions, just large enough to introduce a small camera and some surgical instruments. Most important, it avoids the need to open the abdominal cavity. But does it do the job as well?

Until now, however, surgeons were worried that the keyhole operation might not expose enough of the abdominal cavity and could possibly leave some tumor undetected, or that it might disturb some unnoticed tumor cells in the area and cause them to spread. Earlier studies had reported more cancer recurrences after laparoscopic than open surgery.

HERE'S WHAT'S NEW

A nationwide study reported in the *New England Journal of Medicine* has shown that the laparoscopy is, in fact, an acceptable option to remove colon cancer. The investigation looked at 872 patients with localized colon cancer who were operated on at 48 different hospitals either by the open method or by laparoscopy. After 3 years, there was no statistically significant difference between the two techniques: Tumors spread in 16 percent of the laparoscopy group and in 18 percent of those who had undergone the traditional surgical procedure. Although the laparoscopic operation took 1 hour longer, these patients required less anesthesia, recovered faster, left the hospital sooner, and needed fewer painkillers later on. The rate of surgical complications or the need for repeat surgery was very similar in both groups. However, and this is important, the open procedure more often detected evidence of unsuspected spread to other organs at the time of the initial surgery.

THE BOTTOM LINE

A key factor in choosing between these two procedures is your operative risk. Someone in whom major surgery poses a greater risk—for example, those who are of an advanced age or who have a coexisting cardiac problem—should choose the laparoscopic route. If I needed such an operation myself, I'd probably opt for the open operation because of its most important advantage: its ability to detect tumor cells that have already spread. This permits whatever treatment is necessary to be started earlier than if you waited for symptoms to appear later on.

WHAT THE DOCTOR ORDERED?

COFFEE SAFETY • The relationship between coffee consumption and cancer has been of particular concern to coffee lovers; the recent reports have been contradictory. Research in the 1980s suggested that coffee is associated with an increased risk of cancer of the pancreas and the urinary bladder. This possible association has led to more intensive investigations of the potential relationship between coffee and other common cancers.

HERE'S WHAT'S NEW • Coffee consumption, though suspect, has not been proved to raise the risk of urinary bladder cancer. Whatever association may exist is probably because smokers drink coffee and cigarette smoking is the most important cause of this cancer.

Earlier findings suggesting that drinking 18 or more cups of coffee a week raises the risk of pancreatic cancer have not been substantiated. The National Epidemiology Branch of the National Cancer Institute examined the link between coffee and pancreatic cancer in 136,593 men and women and found no association between coffee and this malignancy.

Other news about the relationship between coffee and cancer is its protective effect against colon cancer. German researchers believe that a highly active antioxidant in coffee, called methylpyridinium reduces the risk of colon cancer. Espresso-type coffee (both caffeinated and decaffeinated) contains two to three times the amount of this anti-cancer agent. Another study showed that drinking 4 or more cups of coffee a day lowers the incidence of colorectal cancer by 24 percent.

THE BOTTOM LINE • Coffee lovers can relax. The brew has been exonerated as a cause of both pancreatic and bladder cancers and has been shown to protect against colon cancer.

Is There a "Best" Treatment for Prostate Cancer?

THERE ARE THREE MAIN THINGS that can go wrong with your prostate: It can become infected (prostatitis, often treatable with antibiotics); it can enlarge and keep you going to the john all night (a big prostate will never kill you, and its symptoms can be helped by medication or surgery), and finally, the prostate gland can become cancerous.

Given all these potential problems, why did nature "bless" men with a prostate to begin with? I asked 25 consecutive patients if they were aware of the prostate's function. Twenty-three of them had no idea; the two who did were doctors. I can hear you asking, "So what *does* it do?" Well, in its own quiet way, the prostate is what keeps mankind going. It makes and stores seminal fluid that nourishes sperm and forms part of your semen. Without seminal fluid, sperm would have nothing in which to swim and would never reach their target egg.

Cancerous prostate cells multiply uncontrollably. They remain in the gland for a while (no one can predict for how long) and then invade nearby tissues and organs. If untreated, they can break loose and travel to distant parts of the body through the bloodstream or the lymphatic system. So the key to preventing such a cancer from killing you is to find it early and eliminate it while it's still in its original location.

Any man can develop prostate cancer, but some are more vulnerable than others. Here are the more important risk factors.

Age. The average age of prostate cancer patients is 70, but younger men are not immune. Your doctor should begin to look for it when you're 50 (or sooner if you are at special risk).

Family history. If your father or brothers had the disease, you should be carefully and regularly checked.

Race. Prostate cancer is most prevalent among African Americans, least common in Asians and Native Americans, with Caucasians falling somewhere in between.

Diet. Consumption of foods rich in saturated fat predisposes men to this cancer, while a lifetime of eating lots of fruits and vegetables appears to reduce the risk. Tomatoes are especially beneficial because of the lycopene they contain. (For more on lycopene, see page 70.)

Early prostate cancer, before the gland has spread, is usually silent. So you must depend on both the digital rectal exam and the prostate-specific antigen (PSA) blood test to find it. Although there is some debate about the usefulness of or need for measuring the PSA routinely, and at what levels it should be considered abnormal, most doctors, including me, still find the test extremely useful (see page 65).

If the PSA level is persistently elevated, or if the doctor feels a suspicious nodule or lump during the rectal exam, he or she will usually perform a sonogram of the prostate. But in the end (no pun intended), you'll need a biopsy to clarify what the lump means and why the PSA level is elevated. Infection also causes the PSA level to rise, so if yours is high, most doctors will prescribe an antibiotic for a couple of weeks to see if it drops to normal. If it doesn't, a biopsy is usually done.

If the biopsy reveals cancer, it will be *graded*. The pathologist looks at the tissue that's been removed to see how quickly the tumor is likely to grow and spread. The grading system varies with the type of cancer. The Gleason system is used in prostate cancer. It ranges from 2 to 10: The lower the number, the less aggressive the tumor. Prostate cancer is also *staged*—that is, evaluated as to whether it has involved any part of the body outside the prostate. A stage 1 cancer is still entirely confined to the gland; stage 4 has spread mainly to bones, the lungs, and the brain.

Armed with this information, a man must now make a decision about treatment. There are several options, depending on the stage and grade of the cancer, your age and general state of health (whether you can tolerate an operation or have some other life-threatening condition), and your own personal preferences. But let me say this up front: Whatever course is recommended to you, it's a good idea to ask for a second opinion. Many variables are involved, and much is at stake. No doctor worth his or her salt will object to your seeking another specialist's view.

There are four major ways to deal with prostate cancer: watchful waiting, surgery, radiation therapy, or hormonal therapy. In deciding which one, alone or in combination, is best for you, remember that they all have risks or side effects that can have an impact not only on your survival but also on the quality of your life.

Watchful waiting. This option is more popular in Europe than it is in the United States. If the cancer appears to be early, nonaggressive, and still confined to the prostate, some doctors adopt a wait-and-see attitude—especially in older men or those who have some other underlying medical condition that will shorten their lives or with whom the complications of treatment may not be well tolerated. These patients are examined at regular and frequent intervals, their PSA level is monitored, and as long as they remain stable without evidence of progression of the cancer, nothing is done. In my own practice, this is the option of last resort. It carries with it the fear, risk, and possibility that the unattended cancer will spread.

Surgery. If you're well enough to withstand an operation and the cancer has not spread, you can have it surgically removed. Before proceeding, surgeons usually take a sample of the lymph nodes in the area of the prostate to make sure they do not contain any cancer cells. If they do, therapy other than surgery is prescribed.

Potential complications of surgery include pain; impotence; inability to produce semen, leading to dry orgasms; infertility; and urinary incontinence.

There are several surgical techniques available, but the best, in my view, is the nerve-sparing procedure developed at the Johns Hopkins Hospital in Baltimore. When this surgery is successful, the incidence of permanent postoperative impotence is reduced but not eliminated. Viagra (sildenafil) has improved the outlook for men. One tablet taken every day for about 9 months, with or without attempted sexual activity, minimizes erectile dysfunction later on.

Radiation therapy. Radiotherapy, in which high-energy x-rays are directed at the cancerous gland, is an alternative to surgery. Such high-intensity radiation can be administered either from an external source or from radioactive seeds inserted near the tumor. (The latter is called implant radiation, also referred to as brachytherapy.) Some patients receive both forms. Radiation may also be done after surgery to attack any cancer cells that may have been left behind.

External radiation can cause hair loss and red, dry, tender skin in the target area as well as impotence. Internal radiation is less likely to cause impotence but may result in temporary incontinence. Both can lead to excessive fatigue, diarrhea, or frequent and painful urination. The good news is that side effects from both external and internal forms are usually temporary.

Hormonal therapy. Prostate cancer thrives on testosterone, the male hormone. Reducing the testosterone level after surgery or radiation may prevent the cancer from recurring or slow its spread, but it is not a cure. It can be done by surgically removing the testicles that make this hormone (a procedure known as an orchiectomy). However, these days your doctor is more likely to prescribe a drug that prevents the testicles from producing testosterone, such as Lupron (leuprolide) and Zoladex (goserelin); stops the adrenal glands, a secondary source of testosterone, from making it; or blocks the hormone's action, such as Eulexin (flutamide). Sometimes another drug, an anti-androgen, is added to block the effect of any remaining testosterone.

Hormonal therapy tends to cause hot flashes, impotence, and loss of sexual desire.

In addition to these tried-and-true therapies, several new approaches are being investigated, such as monoclonal antibody therapy, a treatment that attacks the malignant cells selectively and spares the surrounding normal tissues. However, this treatment is not yet widely used.

Men with prostate cancer agonize over what treatment to choose.

The smart ones ask for a second opinion. But eventually they must make the final say, after weighing all the side effects and risks. So what's a man to do?

HERE'S WHAT'S NEW

Researchers at the M. D. Anderson Cancer Center Orlando in Florida have eased the dilemma somewhat as to which treatment gives the best long-term results. They studied nearly 3,000 men treated for prostate cancer between 1990 and 1998 to see what effect different forms of therapy had on the PSA levels, a marker for containment of the disease. They found no difference among all the treatments listed above, except that low-dose external radiation alone, rarely used anymore, is not nearly as effective as the others.

THE BOTTOM LINE

If you have been told you have prostate cancer, learn about the various treatment options available to you. Ask about their side effects. Most are short-lived and tolerable (considering the alternative). Decide on the one with which you are most comfortable and stick with it. But the most important news is that no one of them is associated with a better or worse long-term outlook than any of the others, except for low-dose radiation.

Diagnosing Prostate Cancer: Yea or Nay for PSA?

MORE THAN 230,000 CASES of prostate cancer are diagnosed every year in this country, and 30,000 men die from it. It's the second leading cause of cancer death in males, accounting for one in every four malignancies in men.

The prostate gland, which is the size of a walnut, is located below the urinary bladder and in front of the rectum—within easy reach of your doctor's finger. Take advantage of this convenient access route and insist on having your prostate examined digitally at least once a year. Although I am a cardiologist, and most patients consult me primarily for matters of the heart, I include a rectal exam in every routine physical. It would do neither my patient nor me any good if I gave him a clean bill of cardiac health and failed to find a curable prostate cancer.

Most prostate tumors grow very slowly in older men, who often outlive them even if they are not treated. Unfortunately, there's no dependable way to know who needs therapy and who can get away without it. As a result, many receive possibly unnecessary therapy with surgery, radiation, or both; or they're left alone, running the risk of dying from their malignancy.

Prostate cancer is difficult to diagnose because it causes no symptoms early on and may not be detectable in a digital rectal exam. (Ironically, benign enlargement of the gland doesn't threaten your life but makes you miserable urinating night and day.) So for years doctors have been relying on measuring the blood level of prostate-specific antigen (PSA), a protein made by the prostate gland. Its concentration in the blood rises in the presence of prostate cancer. Generally speaking (but not always), the higher the PSA, the more aggressive the tumor. A count of 4 (measured in nanograms per milliliter) has always been considered the upper limit of normal. Although higher readings often reflect cancer, they may also be due to infection or enlargement of the gland. When infection is the culprit, these values return to normal after treatment with antibiotics.

PSA determinations are not only useful in diagnosing prostate cancer but also helpful in assessing how well treatment is working. When prostate cancer has been brought under control, the PSA level drops.

When an elevated PSA is not due to infection or benign enlargement of the gland, the prostate is often biopsied in a search for cancer. A biopsy is expensive, not without complications, and not always accurate. Several tissue samples are usually taken, and even they may not reveal the cancer.

The PSA may not only be falsely high, it may be erroneously low, too, in which case the diagnosis is missed at a time when early intervention might be lifesaving. For these reasons, some doctors have disparaged the test and advised against using it. Although this controversy has been going on for years, it is my impression that most internists and urologists still routinely order a PSA test for most men over the age of 50 (and sometimes younger if there is a strong family history of the disease), and they use their judgment in interpreting the result.

HERE'S WHAT'S NEW

A new study in which the National Cancer Institute participated has rekindled a vigorous debate among doctors as to how to interpret PSA results, as well as whether it is worth doing at all. It revealed that when 4 is used as the cutoff point between normal and abnormal, this test misses 15 percent of tumors, including a few aggressive ones in older men. Some believe that the upper limit of normal should be lowered to 2.5. Others counter, however, that doing so could lead to more false positives, needless biopsies, and unnecessary operations. They also point out that the great majority of the cancers associated with these lower numbers are apt to be slow-growing, especially in older men.

Other doctors, especially in Europe, feel that because prostate cancer is often not aggressive, watchful waiting (I prefer to call it "active surveillance") is the best course to follow in the elderly, most of whom will die of causes other than prostate cancer. They believe that therapy should be withheld until the PSA rises significantly or other symptoms of the cancer develop.

The most recent findings suggest that this is not the right thing to do. According to Swedish researchers, low-grade prostate cancers remain dormant for only about 15 years, after which they become aggressive. They studied 223 men whose average age was 72, all of whom had been diagnosed with slow-growing, early-stage prostate cancer. They tracked these men for an average of 21 years, during which time they examined them regularly but did not treat them. By the time the study ended, the cancer had spread in 39 of the men, and 35 men died of it. The researchers conclude that any man who, in the doctor's opinion, has a good chance of living 15 years or longer should be treated for his prostate cancer, no matter how early or slow-growing it appears to be.

In the final analysis, you (the patient) will have to decide whether to have your PSA tested, if and when to have a biopsy, and whether or not to be treated if it is elevated above whatever value your doctor decides is the upper limit of normal—2.5 or 4.

The relevance of all of the above may be moot because of a new observation reported in the *New England Journal of Medicine*. Doctors at the Massachusetts General Hospital in Boston have found a new approach to evaluating the significance of PSA readings. According to results in 36,000 men followed over a period of 12 years, the *rate* at which the PSA increases (called PSA velocity)—rather than the actual numbers—is what's important. They conclude that a rise of at least 2 points in 1 year indicates an aggressive prostate cancer. One in four men in whom this was observed was dead from prostate cancer within 7 years. The Massachusetts General doctors recommend that PSA screening begin at age 40 and be done annually thereafter. If a trend is observed, doing something about it early can be lifesaving. They give the following example. If the initial reading is 0.6, then 1.4 the next year, and then 2.4, and a year later it is 3.2, the implications are ominous, even though all the numbers fall within the traditionally normal range of 4.

Other research calls into question the relevance of PSA testing altogether. Doctors at the University of Pittsburgh School of Medicine have reported in the *Journal of Urology* that testing prostate tissue (not blood) for a protein known as EPCA may detect the presence of prostate cancer 5 years earlier than the PSA does, and with greater accuracy. Currently, when the PSA is high and causes other than cancer have been ruled out, it is necessary to perform a biopsy. Unfortunately, this procedure is not always reliable, because the needle may miss the actual cancer and the report comes back "normal." In such cases, doctors continue to monitor the PSA, and if it keeps climbing, additional biopsies are performed.

The Pittsburgh researchers believe that measuring the EPCA content of the biopsied material can spare men the inconvenience and stress of repeating the procedure, saving precious time as well. EPCA is a marker protein that appears in the cells of organs that contain cancerous tissue. Its presence indicates the earliest evidence of cancer. When they looked for EPCA in biopsies of glands of men who did not have prostate cancer, there was no EPCA present. However, all those who were harboring the malignancy did contain some of this protein. Thus, even if the needle has missed a small cancer and the biopsy result is reported as "normal," the presence of the EPCA confirms cancer. A multicenter study is now under way to validate these observations. If they are confirmed, prostate cancer diagnoses will be easier to make and will be more accurate, too.

THE BOTTOM LINE

I believe that the PSA is a useful test. I measure it in all men over the age of 50 and consider 4 as the cutoff point. I routinely give antibiotics for 2 weeks to everyone in whom the reading is higher than that, just to be sure it does not reflect prostate infection. If the PSA remains elevated but below 9 or 10, I also obtain the free PSA level—that portion of the PSA not bound to protein. When a cancer is present, the free PSA is low. This can further define the need for a biopsy.

I do not normally test the PSA in men over age 80. I prefer active surveillance. However, I will now be influenced by the new findings that low-grade prostate cancers frequently act up after 15 years, and that anyone likely to live that long should be treated early. I also plan to screen my patients earlier and look for the 2-point rise in PSA described above.

A prostate gland that contains cancer, no matter how small, releases a protein called EPCA that can be identified in the tissue removed during a biopsy even if the actual specimen itself does not contain visible cancer cells. This information can spare the patient repeated biopsies and eliminate a dangerous delay in treatment. Further research is needed to validate this finding, but this appears to be a promising diagnostic tool.

What the Doctor Ordered?

LYCOPENE OR TOMATOES? • Men who eat lots of tomatoes have a lower incidence of prostate cancer, presumably because of a carotene-like substance, called lycopene, that gives tomatoes their red color. Is a lycopene supplement as good as the tomatoes themselves?

HERE'S WHAT'S NEW • A paper in the *Journal of the National Cancer Institute* reports that male rats fed tomato powder that included seeds and skin had less risk of dying from prostate cancer than those fed a diet containing only extracted lycopene. The researchers suggest that men who take lycopene supplements in hopes of preventing prostate cancer may be better off eating tomatoes instead. They emphasize that "tomatoes contain dozens of biologically active substances that may work together better than any one would alone."

These findings are similar to those of a study done a few years ago in which researchers investigated whether beta-carotene was as effective as fruits and vegetables in preventing lung cancer. Some 7,000 heavy smokers were given beta-carotene; another 7,000 received a placebo. To the surprise of the investigators, the beta-carotene actually *increased* the risk of lung cancer by 18 percent.

So the lycopene study is the latest example of the increasing awareness that there is no quick fix for the wholesome ingredients in food. Removing or synthesizing a single component does not offer the same benefits and protection against disease as does the intact product.

THE BOTTOM LINE • If you have prostate cancer, are vulnerable to it, or want to prevent it, eat five to seven servings of tomato products a week rather than just taking lycopene supplements. These should be whole tomatoes or processed—juice, soup, or sauce. There is no harm in also taking lycopene supplements, as long as you consume enough tomatoes.

Can Antibiotics Prevent Stomach Cancer?

ALTHOUGH THE INCIDENCE of stomach cancer is declining, there are still nearly 23,000 new cases every year. The disease is responsible for 12,000 deaths in the United States each year, and it is the fourth most common malignancy worldwide, taking the lives of almost 900,000 people annually, mostly in Eastern Asia and Latin America.

Cancer of the stomach begins in that organ's inner lining and, if untreated, spreads throughout the stomach and penetrates its wall to involve adjacent lymph glands and nearby abdominal structures. The best chance for a cure is to find the cancer early and have the stomach removed.

There is no single cause of stomach cancer, but several risk factors have been identified. These include:

- A family history of the disease
- Stomach polyps (especially when more than one exists and they are larger than 3/4 inch)
- Two types of anemia (megaloblastic and pernicious)
- Previous partial removal of the stomach (a gastrectomy) for any reason, such as for severely bleeding ulcers
- A stomach disorder called atrophic gastritis
- Chronic exposure to certain dusts, molds, fumes, and other toxic environmental agents
- Cigarette smoking
- Dietary factors such as a high-salt diet; long-term high intake of nitrates, which are preservatives found in salted, pickled, or smoked foods; as well as eating too few fruits and leafy, green vegetables
- Infection with *Helicobacter pylori* (*H. pylori*), especially when associated with duodenal ulcers

Although all these risk factors have been suspected for about 50 years, many doctors believe that infection with *H. pylori* is the most important one. This organism is present in the stomachs of as many as 90 percent of people in underdeveloped nations and in 50 percent of those in industrialized countries. It may not cause any symptoms for years. *H. pylori* can be identified by a simple breath, stool, or blood test, and it is easily eradicated by a short course of antibiotics.

HERE'S WHAT'S NEW

Although *H. pylori* heads the list of potential causes of stomach cancer, it has never been proved that eradicating it will actually prevent the malignancy. Now comes a study from China, where the incidence of gastric cancer is among the highest in the world. Researchers there evaluated almost 1,700 male and female carriers of *H. pylori* over 7½ years, hundreds of whom already had precancerous stomach lesions. The subjects were assigned to two groups, one of which received a 2-week course of antibiotics to eradicate the organism; the other was given a dummy pill.

None of the 988 patients who didn't have precancerous lesions to begin with and who received the antibiotic therapy developed stomach cancer, but 6 in the placebo group did. Among the hundreds with precancerous lesions at the onset of the study, 7 in the antibiotic group developed stomach cancer, as compared with 11 in the placebo group. It seems as if it may be too late for antibiotics if there is already some evidence that the cancer has begun.

THE BOTTOM LINE

At the present time, most doctors check for *H. pylori* only in patients with ulcers or persistent symptoms of upper gastrointestinal irritation or inflammation. In last year's edition of *Breakthrough Health*, I recommended that anyone with unexplained bad breath or who is intolerant of aspirin should be tested for the presence of *H. pylori*. But it seems to me that we should be screening *everyone* for *H. pylori*, given that such infection is very common, may be silent, and eradicating it with a simple course of antibiotics may prevent stomach cancer.

Alas, the specter of cost efficiency raises its ugly head, as it so often does whenever the issue of disease prevention comes up. The general consensus at the moment is that the study to which I referred above is not really conclusive and screening everybody routinely would be too expensive. But I test my own patients for *H. pylori* if they have a family history of gastrointestinal tumors or if they've had a gastrectomy or any of the other risk factors listed above.

COLD AND FLU

· · · · · · · · · ·

New Flu Vaccination Guidelines

THE "AUTHORITIES" KEEP CHANGING THEIR MINDS with respect to who should be getting an annual flu shot. Not long ago, it was recommended only for those over 65 or anyone who had the kind of chronic disease that could be dangerously worsened by the flu (serious heart, lung, or kidney problems; cancer; or diabetes). That was it.

But the flu kills 36,000 of us every year and sends 114,000 to the hospital. Furthermore, it can make you miserable, even if it isn't life threatening. So healthy younger patients began asking their doctors why, given the fact that it is so easy to prevent, should they be allowed to develop the flu simply because they weren't likely die from it. More and more of them requested the vaccine despite not officially being qualified to have it. The government finally relented. Now anyone who wants a flu shot can have it when supplies of the vaccine are adequate. The only exceptions are people who are allergic to egg protein or chicken, since these proteins are present in the vaccine.

Although the flu shot is now pretty universal for adults, there has always been less enthusiasm for giving it to kids. I don't really understand why, given the fact that along with pneumonia, flu is among the 10 leading causes of death in children between the ages of 1 and 4 years. During the flu season of 2003 to 2004, the flu killed 142 children under the age of 18. Although asthmatic children at any age are particularly hard hit by the flu, presumably because their lungs are more vulnerable to its complications, fewer than 30 percent of them receive the vaccine. But that has now changed, too.

HERE'S WHAT'S NEW

It is now recommended that all children between 6 months and 2 years of age be vaccinated against the flu—this in addition to shots against polio, mumps, measles, rubella (German measles), *H. influenza* B (not to be confused with the flu), hepatitis B, diphtheria, whooping cough, tetanus, and chickenpox. The Centers for Disease Control and Prevention is also emphasizing the importance of vaccinating anyone who takes care of these children, either at home or at school.

Remember that the injectable flu vaccine is prepared from the killed virus. There is no way that it can give you the flu. This is in contrast to the nasal flu vaccine. Marketed as FluMist, this vaccine contains a live, albeit weakened, influenza vaccine administered as a nasal spray that can infect those whose resistance is low—notably the elderly, anyone with a chronic illness or an impaired immune system, and the very young. Also because FluMist is a live vaccine, anyone who receives it becomes a carrier for at least 21 days and can transmit the flu during that time. So it's essential that they avoid close contact with anyone to whom the vaccine must not be given.

In practical terms, that means that health-care workers should receive the conventional killed vaccine, not FluMist. Adolescents and children between the ages of 5 and 17 who take aspirin should not be given the live nasal vaccine either because, if they develop a viral infection, aspirin makes them vulnerable to Reye's syndrome. FluMist should be used only by healthy people between the ages of 5 and 49.

Pregnant and nursing women who could transmit the infection to their fetuses or children should have the injectable form, not the nasal vaccine. New research indicates an additional and surprising reason for pregnant women to get the vaccine. Researchers at Columbia University in New York City reported to a meeting of the American Psychiatric Association that children born to women who contract the flu during the first half of their pregnancy appear to have an increased risk of becoming schizophrenic later in life. If they were infected with the flu during the first trimester, the risk of this mental illness was increased sevenfold; exposure during the first half of pregnancy raised it three times. It's not clear how the flu virus predisposes to schizophrenia, but it's thought to be due to brain chemicals released by the presence of the virus.

THE BOTTOM LINE

Everyone should be vaccinated against the flu, including kids between the ages of 6 months and 2 years, as well as pregnant women. There appears to be a link between a pregnant woman developing the flu and the risk of her child having schizophrenia. The nasal flu vaccine (FluMist), though effective, should be taken only by healthy people between the ages of 5 and 49 years and not by pregnant women. Unlike the injectable vaccine that is made from dead viruses, FluMist contains a weakened but live virus that can cause infection in those who are vulnerable or can be passed from a mother to her unborn child.

DEPRESSION

· · · · · · · · · ·

Be Careful with Antidepressants

AN ESTIMATED 19 MILLION AMERICAN ADULTS are depressed for any number of reasons. They may have lost someone dear to them; they may have seemingly unsolvable economic problems; they may be disappointed in love; or they may have been exposed to some severe stress such as the September 11 attacks (post-traumatic stress disorder). The list is as inexhaustible as life itself. But there are also many individuals who have no apparent reason to be down in the dumps and don't know why they are. Sometimes they're anxious and not depressed, but these two emotions often go hand in hand, and it is not always clear which is the dominant one.

Doctors have been treating depressed patients ever since one person confided to another how he or she feels. In addition to professional and family support, successive generations of drugs have become available to lift one's mood. They are more widely prescribed and used these days than ever before.

The current generation of antidepressants are called selective serotonin reuptake inhibitors (SSRIs), the best known and most widely used of which currently are Prozac (fluoxetine), Paxil (paroxetine), Zoloft (sertraline), Celexa (citalopram), Lexapro (escitalopram), and Luvox (fluvoxamine). Two other commonly prescribed antidepressants, Effexor (venlafaxine) and Serzone (nefazodone), are closely related to the SSRIs but have fewer side effects. All of these medications ease depression by increasing the concentration of a brain chemical called serotonin, too little of which is believed to contribute to depression.

Two other effective and popular antidepressants—Remeron (mirtazapine) and Wellbutrin (bupropion)—work by a different, unknown mechanism.

As many as 10 percent of kids and teenagers are so seriously depressed that some 2,000 of them between the ages 10 and 19 commit suicide every year. Almost 2 million more try it but don't succeed. Last year, there were almost 11 million prescriptions dispensed to depressed boys and girls younger than 18.

HERE'S WHAT'S NEW

Despite the fact that there is no new evidence that antidepressants have resulted in childhood suicide, the concern persists. (As I indicated in last year's edition of *Breakthrough Health,* Prozac is the only antidepressant approved for children.)

Although most psychopharmacologists and the psychiatrists prescribing antidepressants for kids are convinced that the drugs have actually resulted in *fewer* suicides, the FDA generally supports an advisory panel's conclusion that antidepressants sometimes raise the risk of suicidal behavior in youth. In fact, there is now concern that adults, as well as children, may be vulnerable, too. It's a hard call because one is never sure what leads a depressed person to suicide—the underlying emotional disturbance itself or its aggravation by treatment with these drugs. The FDA is continuing to accumulate data and has requested that the manufacturers of all the antidepressants listed above label their products with a suicide warning.

Until all the evidence is in, if you are taking one of these drugs or know someone who is, and you have noted a recent change in thinking or behavior, such as suicidal thoughts, hostility, anxiety, or difficulty sleeping, let your doctor know immediately. These drugs must be withdrawn gradually and under the guidance of the prescribing physician; do not stop them abruptly or on your own.

THE BOTTOM LINE

Depression is an ongoing problem for millions of children and adults. In addition to personal and professional support, antidepressants can help. But be aware that some specialists and the FDA fear that these drugs can also worsen depression to the point of suicide. Be especially careful about giving these antidepressants to children for whom Prozac is the only approved drug in this category. Whatever your age and regardless of which antidepressant you're taking, if you need to discontinue it for any reason, taper it; do not stop it abruptly.

Fish Oil Benefits

SCIENTISTS HAVE KNOWN for some time that populations with the highest consumption of fish have the lowest rates of depression. According to one study, English women who eat very little fish while pregnant are at twice the risk of becoming depressed after their babies are born than those who eat fish regularly.

HERE'S WHAT'S NEW

These and similar observations are substantiated by some very promising animal experiments. For example, 18 days after piglets were fed omega-3 fatty acids, their brains contained higher levels of the neurotransmitter serotonin in the frontal cortex (where depression and impulsivity are regulated). Similar findings were observed in other studies in which animals were given the antidepressant Prozac (fluoxetine). (Docosahexaenoic acid, or DHA, is the omega-3 fatty acid with the most direct influence on brain development and function.)

Trials using omega-3 fatty acids in humans have been conducted in England and in the United States. At the University of Sheffield in Great Britain, 70 depressed patients who had not been helped by serotonin reuptake inhibitors such as Prozac were given omega-3 fatty acids. After 12 weeks, 69 percent of them showed marked improvement compared with 25 percent of those who received placebos. Researchers at Massachusetts General Hospital in Boston who conducted an omega-3 clinical trial believe that these treatments have definite promise.

Preliminary studies suggest that 1 gram a day of omega-3 fatty acids is effective, whether by taking a nutritional supplement available at most health food stores or simply by eating cold-water fish such as salmon, sardines, or tuna several times a week. Because omega-3 trials have been so successful against depression, researchers are hopeful that omega-3 will also help patients with schizophrenia, bipolar disorder, and violent behavior.

THE BOTTOM LINE

Omega-3 fatty acids, from fish or capsule supplements, promise to be effective in treating depression. A dose of 1 gram a day may be all you need.

DIABETES

· · · · · · · · · ·

How to Recognize Pre-diabetes

IF YOU EVER DOUBT the importance of diabetes, look at these numbers: 18 million Americans already have the disease, and 80 percent of them will eventually develop its complications, the most important and common of which are vascular disease of the heart, brain, kidneys, eyes, and blood vessels throughout the body. To reduce the chances of suffering these consequences or to delay their onset, doctors emphasize the importance of maintaining stringent sugar control and modifying any risk factors for the disease that may be present. These include overweight, abnormal cholesterol levels, smoking, high blood pressure, and physical inactivity.

We are in the midst of a diabetes epidemic. There are almost 1.5 million new cases every year in this country alone (up from 900,000 just 5 years ago). Adult diabetes (type 2) is striking more and more *children* than ever before; it will leave almost 25,000 Americans blind this year alone and require more than 100,000 people with diabetes to either undergo dialysis or have a kidney transplant and 82,000 to have a toe, foot, or leg amputated. In addition to all this suffering, diabetes imposes a staggering financial burden of $132 billion annually, expected to reach $192 billion by the year 2020.

There are two major types of diabetes, each with totally different causes. However, they both result in high blood sugar and similar long-term complications. Type 1 (also called juvenile diabetes because it usually begins early in life) results from the gradual destruction of insulin-producing beta cells in the pancreas by an abnormally functioning autoimmune system. Insulin is the hormone that makes it possible for the body to convert glucose to body energy. When it's lacking, the unused glucose accumulates in the blood and its level rises.

Patients with type 2 diabetes also have high blood sugar but for a different reason. Although their pancreatic cells do make insulin, it doesn't get into the body's cells to allow them to break down glucose to provide energy. As a result, the glucose (sugar) level in the blood rises. This inability to utilize insulin is most likely to occur in people who are overweight and don't exercise. Why some of them develop diabetes and others don't remains a mystery, although there is probably some genetic basis for it.

The two forms of diabetes are treated differently. Every patient with type 1 *must* receive insulin because his or her body does not produce it. Because people with type 2 diabetes do make enough insulin, at least early in the course of their disease, the aim of therapy is to overcome the body's resistance to this hormone. (As the disease progresses, the insulin-producing pancreatic cells, having tried and tried to correct matters by making more and more insulin, finally become exhausted and don't make enough. At this point, some people with type 2 need insulin, too.)

The period of insulin resistance before frank diabetes sets in is referred to as the pre-diabetic state. We used to consider a fasting blood sugar of more than 110 milligrams per deciliter as reflecting pre-diabetes. Recommended treatment for pre-diabetes has always been weight reduction and exercise.

HERE'S WHAT'S NEW

As a result of ongoing data analysis, it is now estimated that there are 41 million pre-diabetics among us. According to new guidelines from the American Diabetes Association, the upper limit for normal fasting blood sugar has been dropped from 110 to 100. If your reading is below 100, you're fine; between 100 and 125, you are pre-diabetic; a fasting sugar higher than 125 indicates diabetes.

A glucose tolerance test will define your category more accurately. After you've fasted for 12 hours, your doctor draws blood and tests the sugar level, then you drink a measured amount of glucose. For the next 4 hours, while you're sitting in the waiting room reading last year's magazines, your blood is drawn every half hour to measure its sugar content. If it climbs to between 140 and 199 at the 2-hour mark, you are pre-diabetic.

Most people with pre-diabetes go on to develop full-blown type 2 diabetes within 10 years. But they can usually delay or prevent that from happening if they lose 5 to 7 percent of their body weight (10 to 15 pounds if they started off at about 200 pounds). That's best done by a combination of diet and exercise.

People with pre-diabetes, though usually symptom-free, are more vulnerable to heart disease. In addition to their high blood sugar, pre-diabetic men usually have a waist measurement of at least 40 inches; in women it's at least 35 inches. They also have other danger signals such as a high triglyceride level, low HDL (the "good" cholesterol), high LDL (the "bad" cholesterol), and a blood pressure reading higher than 130/85. All of these risk factors should be corrected.

Who should get a fasting blood sugar test to see if they are pre-diabetic? In my own practice, I have it done annually in everyone, male or female, over the age of 45—or younger if they are overweight or have a family history of diabetes, high blood pressure, elevated LDL, low HDL, and high triglycerides, especially if they are African American or Hispanic.

If you have pre-diabetes, you can reduce your risk of it developing further by 58 percent if you lose weight through diet (low in fat, low in calories) and exercise (30 minutes of brisk walking every day). At the same time, you must quit smoking, normalize your blood pressure if it's high, and optimize your cholesterol profile, preferably with one of the statin drugs, such as Lipitor (atorvastatin) or Zocor (simvastatin).

Although these are the most effective interventions, if they don't result in the necessary weight loss for whatever reason, you can try taking sugar-lowering drugs, such as Glucophage (metformin). However, the FDA has not approved either of these drugs specifically for this purpose. Discuss with your doctor whether you should use them.

More recently, doctors from Israel's Tel Aviv University published in the journal *Circulation* their experience with bezafibrate, a drug that lowers both cholesterol and triglycerides. Bezafibrate was found to decrease the risk of developing diabetes by 30 percent. This drug is not sold in the United States, but two medications with similar action—Lopid (gemfibrozil) and Tricor (fenofibrate) are available.

THE BOTTOM LINE

Type 2 diabetes, the most common kind by far, develops gradually. There is a pre-diabetic state that can often be diagnosed by measuring the fasting blood sugar. You should have it done if you're over 45, especially if you're overweight or have a family history of diabetes.

If you are found to be pre-diabetic, you can reduce your risk of developing the full-blown disease by losing weight and exercising.

Remember that someone with pre-diabetes is vulnerable to heart disease. So it's also important to normalize all your other risk factors. In addition to overweight, these include your cholesterol profile, smoking, and blood pressure. If you lose the extra pounds, you have a much better chance of not becoming diabetic. Several drugs can also help if you cannot achieve the necessary weight loss.

ACE Inhibitor Benefits

THE LEADING CAUSE OF DEATH in people with diabetes is vascular disease—heart attacks and stroke, blindness, kidney failure, and amputations of the lower limbs whose blood supply has been reduced by blockages in their arteries. A person with diabetes is twice as likely to die from heart trouble than is someone with a normal blood sugar.

HERE'S WHAT'S NEW

Researchers at the University of Alberta in Canada have found that when someone who is newly diagnosed with diabetes starts taking an ACE inhibitor and continues to do so indefinitely, his or her risk of death from all causes is cut in half, and death from heart disease alone drops by 23 percent. This is true regardless of whether any of these individuals already have evidence of heart disease when they start taking the drug.

ACE stands for angiotensin converting enzyme. ACE inhibitors—of which the prototypes are Capoten (captopril), Vasotec (enalapril), and Altace (ramipril)—block the action of angiotensin, a natural enzyme in the body that narrows, or constricts, blood vessels and raises blood pressure. It is also believed to play a role in the development of heart disease. ACE inhibitors are therefore commonly used to treat elevated pressure and to exert a beneficial action on heart muscle. By relaxing the arteries, these medications increase the blood flow to the heart and slow the development of heart disease (independent of their blood-pressure-lowering effect).

THE BOTTOM LINE

If you have diabetes, and especially if it was recently diagnosed, ask your doctor about adding an ACE inhibitor to your treatment regimen—regardless of whether or not your blood pressure is high. These new data from Canada suggest that this can prolong your life. One word of caution: A small number of people who take these drugs develop a dry cough. If that happens, tell your doctor about it. He or she can take you off the ACE inhibitor and replace it with an angiotensin receptor blocker (ARB). This group of drugs acts essentially the same as the ACE inhibitors but does not cause a cough.

Reduce Your Risk of Diabetes with Coffee

THERE HAS NEVER BEEN ANY REASON to tie coffee to diabetes, except when sugar is added to it. So I can't imagine what motivated researchers to look for a link between diabetes and coffee intake.

HERE'S WHAT'S NEW

A host of recent findings indicates that long-term regular coffee intake reduces the risk of type 2 (the adult form) diabetes. It's not clear what does the protecting—the caffeine or one or more of the many other ingredients in the brew such as its antioxidants or minerals like magnesium. But whatever it is, the *Journal of the American Medical Association* has reported the results of a survey conducted among more than 7,000 men and an equal number of women. Drinking 3 to 4 cups of coffee a day reduced the risk of developing diabetes by 29 percent. The larger the amount consumed, the greater this benefit.

In women who drink at least 10 cups a day, that risk is reduced by an average of 79 percent; in men, it falls by 55 percent. This salutary effect may also reflect the fact that coffee increases energy expenditure, which may result in some weight loss, and weight loss is good for people with diabetes.

If coffee appears to prevent diabetes, you would think that those who already have diabetes should be drinking it. A recent small study done by researchers at Duke University Medical Center in Durham, North Carolina, suggests just the opposite! They found that taking caffeine at mealtime increases sugar levels and reduces insulin sensitivity among people with type 2 (the adult form) of diabetes. Interestingly, coffee consumption does not affect fasting sugar readings, only those following a meal. The researchers believe that their findings are important enough to advise people with diabetes who regularly drink caffeinated beverages to *reduce or eliminate their intake*, especially at mealtime and particularly if they are having trouble controlling their blood sugar level.

THE BOTTOM LINE

Drinking coffee (but without added sugar) lowers your chances of developing diabetes. But once you have the disease, you may be better off reducing your intake or eliminating it altogether.

Sugar or Spice—Which One Is Nice?

TO PREVENT AND CORRECT the body's resistance to insulin, people with diabetes and those prone to it must lose weight by means of diet and exercise. Dropping only a few pounds increases the effectiveness of insulin. (Even someone in a pre-diabetic state, the latest definition of which is a fasting blood sugar as low as 100 milligrams per deciliter—see page 82—can prevent the disease from progressing by losing enough weight.) Easily digested junk foods such as chips and nondiet soft drinks should be avoided because they require larger amounts of insulin, which simply doesn't work in these people. Exercise is important because working muscles draw more glucose out of the bloodstream and increase the efficiency of insulin.

If you are overweight and frankly diabetic (as opposed to being pre-diabetic), and you can't or won't lose weight, there are several drugs available to lower your blood sugar. They do so by either making the body less resistant to insulin or forcing the pancreas to make even more insulin. However, no drug is as effective as weight reduction in the long run. Furthermore, there's no evidence that lowering blood sugar with any of these drugs is effective in preventing the long-term complications of diabetes. These medications should never be considered as primary treatment.

There are five classes of oral sugar-lowering drugs.

- Sulfonylureas—the most recent widely used in this category are Glucotrol (glipizide), Glynase (glyburide), and Amaryl (glimepiride)—usually lower blood sugar by about 20 percent. They do so by increasing the amount of insulin secreted by the pancreas.

- Biguinides, such as Glucophage (metformin), are especially effective in overweight people with diabetes and often prevent the disease in those with pre-diabetes. They increase the effectiveness of insulin and reduce the amount of glucose in the blood by blocking its release from the liver. In so doing, they lower the risk of pre-diabetics developing the disease by 30 percent (see page 85). Unlike sulfonylureas, biguinides do not stimulate insulin production, but they do reduce resistance to it.

- Alpha-glucosidase inhibitors, such as Precose (acarbose) and Glyset (miglitol), prevent stomach enzymes from converting starch and other complex carbohydrates you eat into simple sugars. This stops them from being absorbed and entering the bloodstream. These drugs are useful for treating both types of diabetes.

• Thiazolidinediones, such as Avandia (rosiglitazone) and Actos (pioglitazone), lower insulin resistance by acting on muscle, fat, and the liver so that they decrease the production of glucose and improve how it's used. Their mechanism of action is not clear. Earlier versions of these drugs were withdrawn from the market because they caused liver damage. Although the new ones are better in that regard, if you take either of them, you should nevertheless have your blood tested regularly to monitor the health of your liver.

• Meglitidines, such as Prandin (repaglinide) and Starlix (nateglinide), lower blood sugar by stimulating the pancreas to release more insulin. Unlike the sulfonylureas, however, these drugs work only when glucose levels are high.

HERE'S WHAT'S NEW

A new and interesting observation has been made about a common kitchen-cabinet spice that may lower blood sugar levels and stave off the onset of type 2 diabetes in people who have pre-diabetes. It sounds almost too good to be true. Researchers at the Beltsville Human Nutrition Research Center in Maryland found that as little as $1/2$ teaspoon of cinnamon a day can reduce blood glucose by up to 30 percent and at the same time decrease cholesterol and other fats in the blood—presumably by increasing sensitivity to insulin. Add a little spice to your life every day with $1/2$ teaspoon of cinnamon in your tea, coffee, cereal, or whatever. Then check your blood sugar level after a month or so to see if it has made a difference. Tell your doctor (and me) about it. I'd love to know if it works for you.

On another note, if you have type 2 diabetes and are taking one of the thiazolidinediones mentioned above (Avandia, Actos), you should be aware that recent research suggests that they may increase the risk of heart failure in some patients by about 70 percent. If you have any degree of heart failure or any cardiac condition that leaves you vulnerable to it, discuss the use of these drugs with your doctor. If you develop any evidence or symptoms of heart failure while you're on one of them, either reduce the dose or, preferably, switch to some other therapy.

THE BOTTOM LINE

Unlike type 1 diabetes, in which the pancreas does not make enough insulin, people with type 2 diabetes have enough insulin but are resistant to it. The best way to deal with that is to lose weight. Adding $1/2$ teaspoon of cinnamon to what you eat or drink every day may also help lower your blood sugar and cholesterol levels. It's worth a try.

There are five main types of oral medications for treating type 2 diabetes if weight loss alone isn't enough, each with its own mode of action. Actos and Avandia lower blood sugar in different ways but can increase the risk of heart failure by 70 percent, especially in someone with a heart condition. If you have any heart problem, you may be better off taking another drug, or even insulin, to lower your blood sugar.

DIARRHEA

• • • • • • • • •

Breakthrough Drug Avenges Montezuma

IT'S ESTIMATED THAT 20 to 50 percent of all international travelers, roughly 10 million people, develop diarrhea every year. Those visiting any area in the world where hygiene and sanitation leave something to be desired (Africa, Asia, Central and South America) are at particularly high risk. Nothing will spoil a vacation or a business trip like spending most of it on the john. Travelers' diarrhea goes by a variety of names, the most common of which is "the runs." If you happen to be in Mexico, you might hear it referred to as the Mexican Two-Step or Montezuma's Revenge.

Travelers' diarrhea has many different causes. Most cases are caused by the common bowel bacterium *Escherichia coli* (*E. coli*), whose strains vary in different parts of the world. From time to time, the diarrhea is due to a parasite or to dysentery, both of which are apt to be more serious and persistent than the run-of-the-mill *E. coli* variety, which usually is contracted by consuming contaminated food or water. That's because even if you toe the line and do your best to avoid any suspicious food, you're at the mercy of cooks and food handlers who carry the germs on their hands because they don't bother to wash them (despite the pleas posted in restaurant washrooms for them to do so).

The usual symptoms of travelers' diarrhea are frequent watery bowel movements accompanied by abdominal cramps, nausea or vomiting, loss of appetite, and a low-grade fever. Symptoms usually last only a few days, and most people recover without specific treatment. However, if you're sick for longer than a week, have your stool tested to find out what organism is causing it.

Here's the best ways to avoid traveler's diarrhea.

- Don't drink tap water or even brush your teeth with it.

- Drink bottled water or carbonated beverages, but only after making sure that the seal on the bottle is intact. (Boiled tea and coffee are safe.)

- Don't add ice to your drinks.

- Don't have unpasteurized milk or dairy products.

- Don't eat raw fruits or vegetables. If they can be peeled, do so yourself.

- Avoid leafy raw vegetables such as spinach and cut-up fruit salad.

- Do not eat raw or rare meat or fish (even in Japan). Food should be served hot and meat well cooked.

- Don't eat food from street vendors.

- Don't swim in streams, lakes, or pools.

- Before you eat, clean your hands, preferably with prepackaged hand wipes or antiseptic gel—not tap water.

Take along some Imodium (loperamide) or Lomotil (diphenoxylate and atropine), as well as an antiseptic hand gel. Although you probably won't need an antibiotic, bring some Cipro (ciprofloxacin), too, in case the diarrhea persists and is accompanied by high fever and blood in the stool. However, if the diarrhea continues after 3 days of taking the Cipro, consult a doctor.

One of the biggest problems with ongoing diarrhea is dehydration, especially in kids and the elderly. You can prevent dehydration by drinking lots of purified water or other clear liquids such as juices and soft drinks to compensate for the water you're losing. It's a good idea to take along a few packs of commercially available "oral rehydration" mix. Add water to the powder, which contains a balance of minerals that can be depleted by the diarrhea.

HERE'S WHAT'S NEW

The FDA has recently approved rifaximin (marketed as Xifaxan), an antibiotic that, according to its proponents, promises to "change the way we manage traveler's diarrhea." Rifaximin belongs to a class of drugs that is not absorbed but remains in the gastrointestinal tract where it kills harmful bacteria (unlike other antibiotics such as Cipro that are absorbed into the bloodstream). As a result, there is little likelihood of developing resistance to it.

In tests of U.S. students visiting Mexico for 2 weeks, 85 percent of those who took rifaximin remained free of diarrhea as compared with only 49 percent of those on placebos. Although Cipro is very effective, many doctors believe it should be reserved for life-threatening illnesses, especially since overuse can allow harmful bacteria to become immune to it.

THE BOTTOM LINE

Preventing traveler's diarrhea is mostly a matter of good hygiene. However, quite often despite all your best efforts, you will become sick. Although there are several effective antibiotics to kill the offending bacteria, a new one on the horizon can prevent the infection.

EAR INFECTIONS

• • • • • • • • • •

Try Pain Relief before Antibiotics

I HAVE IMPECCABLE CREDENTIALS for dispensing advice on how to treat children's earaches, not only as a doctor but also as a father of four and a grandfather of seven. Anyone who has raised or lived with infants and children is familiar with the scenario. The child awakes crying, holding an ear, and often has a fever. After a sleepless night for all concerned, a decision about antibiotics has to be made. Traditionally, that has always been the route to go, along with some acetaminophen or a nonsteroidal anti-inflammatory such as ibuprofen to reduce the pain. When you call the pediatrician, for whom such calls constitute the majority of his or her telephone consultations, you're usually reassured that a trip to the office is unnecessary. (You were smart enough not to ask for a house call!) After 2 or 3 days, the earache (doctors call it acute otitis media) subsides, with or without the antibiotic—until the next time.

Heretofore, pediatricians have usually prescribed antibiotics in such situations, more likely to assuage the parents' anxiety than because it was really necessary. This time-honored approach to what is one of the most common childhood ailments (in the year 2000 there were 16 million office visits and 13 million antibiotic prescriptions written for ear infections) has recently been questioned and revised because of the emergence of growing numbers of antibiotic-resistant bacteria. The worry is that if kids are given antibiotics often enough when they don't really need them, their bodies may fail to respond to them during some future serious infection such as pneumonia or meningitis.

HERE'S WHAT'S NEW

Pediatricians have come out with new guidelines for treating ear infections in children. They emphasize that you should relieve the child's pain first and not rush to give antibiotics that neither lessen pain nor reduce fever any more quickly than do painkillers in the first 24 hours. What's more, 80 percent of these infections clear up without antibiotics anyway.

So here's the official recommendation of the American Academy of Pediatrics and the American Academy of Family Physicians. If your child has an earache, treat the pain with ibuprofen or acetaminophen in the first 24 hours. If your child is more than 2 years old and the symptoms are not severe, wait for 2 or 3 days before starting an antibiotic (however, pediatricians usually prescribe antibiotics right away for children between the ages of 6 months and 2 years who have severe symptoms). If antibiotics do become necessary, then amoxicillin is the one doctors usually prescribe.

Let me share with you some new information about earaches in kids. Doctors at the Christian Medical College in India compared the effectiveness of povidone-iodine—the antiseptic scrub that surgeons use to wash their hands before operating—and eardrops of the antibiotic Cipro (ciprofloxacin) in 40 children with chronic ear infections. Half the kids were given 3 drops of povidone-iodine solution in their ears; the others received 3 drops of Cipro, both three times a day for 10 days. The youngsters were checked every week for 4 weeks. The doctors found both treatments equally effective. However, povidone-iodine is far less expensive and doesn't carry with it the potential problem of drug resistance. They conclude that it can effectively treat ear infections and should be considered an alternative to antibiotic therapy. It's something to discuss with your child's pediatrician.

THE BOTTOM LINE

If your child is over 2 years of age and develops an earache, don't rush to get an antibiotic unless there is high fever and the kid is obviously very sick. First try a painkiller such as a pediatric dose of acetaminophen or a nonsteroidal anti-inflammatory drug such as ibuprofen for a day or two. If symptoms persist or worsen, or if the fever climbs, the doctor may prescribe amoxicillin. The reason for this conservative approach is that 80 percent of these infections clear up by themselves after a couple of days, and the indiscriminate use of antibiotics can and indeed has resulted in the appearance of antibiotic-resistant strains of bacteria that make treating serious infection later on more difficult. Povidone-iodine drops in the affected ears appear to work as well as topical antibiotics.

ENDOMETRIOSIS

• • • • • • • • • •

Two New Options for Pain Relief

MORE THAN 5.5 MILLION American girls and women of reproductive age have endometriosis, a disorder in which tissue that normally lines the cavity of the uterus (the endometrium) appears in other locations, where it has no right to be. Some research indicates that the disorder affects more Asians than Caucasians or African Americans.

In a woman with endometriosis, endometrial tissue has most commonly migrated to the ovaries (in 75 percent of cases), or to the fallopian tubes (along which eggs travel from the ovaries to the uterus), or elsewhere in the pelvis. But it is sometimes found between the rectum and vagina or in the rectum itself, in the appendix, in the urinary bladder, and occasionally in the stomach. It has even very rarely been present in the gallbladder, spleen, liver, and lungs. Symptoms (mainly pain, bleeding, and infertility) usually become apparent soon after the onset of menstrual periods, and the disorder comes and goes until menopause.

The wandering endometrial tissue, wherever it happens to end up and by whatever route it got there, sometimes behaves as if it were still in the uterus. In other words, it can menstruate! That's why symptoms of endometriosis are usually intermittent, and their timing is often related to the normal menstrual period. No two women with endometriosis have exactly the same complaint because their symptoms depend on the location of the misplaced uterine tissue. Unlike normal menstruating tissue in the uterus, wandering endometrial tissue has no way of being shed as it is from the uterus every month. It remains in its location, where it eventually forms scar tissue and adhesions that irritate the area, causing symptoms not only during the menstrual period but all month long.

Why endometrial tissue wanders in this way is not fully understood. There may be a genetic basis to it. If your sister or mother has it, there's a greater chance that you will, too. Many gynecologists believe, however, that this disorder is mainly due to an abnormal immune system that allows these cells not only to migrate from the uterus but also to survive where they don't belong.

There is no cure for endometriosis, but there are ways to reduce the pain it causes, restore fertility, and shrink the size of the "lost" tissue. However, the best long-term treatment option is to remove the offending tissue *if possible*.

Managing endometriosis first and foremost involves pain relief. This is best done with aspirin, nonsteroidal anti-inflammatory drugs (NSAIDs), and acetaminophen. The sooner you start taking them when you have pain, the more effective they are. If the pain is very severe, you may need a prescription-strength painkiller.

Any drug or hormone (such as progestin) that stops menstrual periods will also ease the symptoms of endometriosis. This, however, is not a satisfactory long-term solution for many women. Progestin is not as popular as it once was, because the high doses required result in bloating, weight gain, depression, and irregular vaginal bleeding. It may also sometimes cause a prolonged and negative effect on ovarian function even after it has been stopped.

Other popular treatments are the gonadotropin-releasing hormone (GnRH) agonists that decrease the brain's production of luteinizing hormones (LH) and follicle-stimulating hormones (FSH). (LH and FSH stimulate the formation of estrogen, the hormone that promotes growth of endometrial tissue.) GnRH agonists take about a month to work and are available as a nasal spray or as a monthly injection. Pregnant women should not use them.

HERE'S WHAT'S NEW

A team of Italian gynecologists in Milan treated 50 women with endometriosis by having them take oral contraceptives *continuously* without the usual 1-week pause. This ensured that there were no menstrual periods during which pain could occur. After 2 years, 80 percent of the women reported that they were satisfied with the treatment and that it had resulted in less pain. According to the president-elect of the American Society of Reproductive Medicine, "if women suffering from endometriosis are not ready to become pregnant, continuous oral contraceptive use is one of the better ways to manage pain. The effect of the Pill is reversible, so future fertility is possible, and if side effects (of the Pill) are more troublesome than warranted by pain relief, it can be easily discontinued. For these reasons, oral contraceptives are an excellent option" for the management of the symptoms of endometriosis.

There is no downside to taking the Pill continuously to suppress menstruation. The FDA has just approved Seasonale (ethinyl estradiol/levenorgestrel), a contraceptive pill that allows women to have just four menstrual periods a year.

Another promising approach to reducing the pain of endometriosis is one of the aromatase inhibitors used in the treatment of advanced breast cancer (see page 42). In a small study done at Northwestern University Feinberg School of Medicine in Chicago, researchers found that 10 premenopausal women with painful endometriosis who had previously not responded to any other therapy experienced dramatic improvement in their symptoms after taking an aromatase inhibitor. In this case, the drug used was Femara (letrozole), one of several in this class. There were no significant side effects or complications during a 6-month period.

THE BOTTOM LINE

If you are troubled by ongoing pain, bleeding, and cramps from endometriosis, and you cannot be treated surgically, you should consider going on the Pill and taking it nonstop—that is, without the customary week off once a month. When you want to begin trying to have a baby, you simply stop the Pill.

Another alternative for controlling the pain of endometriosis that's worth exploring with your doctor is an aromatase inhibitor called Femara. Results of a small study of premenopausal women with pain not responsive to other medication suggest that it's worth a try. Side effects and complications from its use appear to be minimal.

EPILEPSY

· · · · · · · · ·

New Guidelines for New Drugs

EPILEPSY IS A NEUROLOGICAL DISORDER in which electrical signals in the brain go haywire. The result is an entire spectrum of seizures ranging from a glassy-eyed stare to jerking movements, generalized convulsions, and loss of consciousness. The extent and severity of these seizures depend on how much of the brain is involved. About 2.5 million people in the United States and 40 million worldwide have this disorder. Most are adults over age 65 and children, but it can occur at any age. Five to 10 percent of Americans will suffer at least one seizure during their lifetime; in 30 percent they will recur. When first diagnosed, this condition is called new-onset epilepsy.

The cause of epilepsy is never determined in about 70 percent of those who suffer from it. In the remaining 30 percent, it's the result of a head injury, an infection such as meningitis, a brain tumor, a complication of brain surgery, stroke, Alzheimer's disease, or hardening of the brain arteries so that not enough blood is flowing to various parts of the brain.

Regardless of the underlying cause, many different triggers can set off a seizure in someone with epilepsy. These include stress, lack of sleep, starvation, dehydration, infection, flashing lights, medications, and high fever (especially in children).

For many years, there was only a handful of drugs available to control epileptic seizures. The best known among them are phenobarbital, phenytoin, carbamazepine, and valproic acid. They are fairly inexpensive, and they work in many people who have used them for as long as 30 years. However, there are many patients in whom they do not effectively control seizures but who continue to take them because they are resigned to their fate and are unaware of the new treatments available to them. These older medications occasionally cause serious side effects, too. For example, phenobarbital is a sedative that leaves you chronically tired; phenytoin can affect the gums.

There are three categories of *refractory* epilepsy in which medications do not prevent seizures: (1) partial, in which the seizures affect only one area of the brain; (2) generalized, in which the entire brain is involved; and (3) the Lennox-Gastaut syndrome, characterized by mixed seizures.

HERE'S WHAT'S NEW

Seven new drugs have been approved during the past 10 years to treat epilepsy, providing patients with long-needed alternatives. In order to make doctors and patients alike aware of them, specialists from the American Academy of Neurology and the American Epilepsy Society have for the first time in 10 years issued new guidelines for the treatment of the various forms of epilepsy.

Four of the new drugs are especially effective in teens and adults with new-onset epilepsy. They are Neurontin (gabapentin), Lamictal (lamotrigine), Trileptal (oxcarbazepine), and Topamax (topiramate). These medications are used one at a time, not in combination with each other. Lamictal is also recommended for children who have been recently diagnosed with absence seizures (also known as petit mal seizures).

If your child has refractory partial epilepsy and has continued to have seizures, any one of the four new drugs listed above will help. Discuss with your doctor whether they should replace or be added to your current treatment. For adults with refractory partial epilepsy, the new anti-epileptic drugs may have to be taken in combination.

For generalized epilepsy that has not responded to older therapy, Topamax is likely to be the most effective drug. For the drop seizures (loss of muscle control resulting in physical collapse) associated with Lennox-Gastaut syndrome, Lamictal and Topamax are recommended.

THE BOTTOM LINE

Although these guidelines are primarily for doctors, I am drawing your attention to them so that you may discuss them with your doctor or obtain a second opinion if necessary. The authors of these guidelines emphasize that it is extremely important to select the right drug with which to start treatment when epileptic attacks first occur. Doing so can continue to have a major beneficial impact for years and years.

EYE PROBLEMS

When Tears Are Not Enough

AN ESTIMATED 10 MILLION AMERICANS suffer from dry eyes either because their production of tears has decreased or because their quality deteriorated. Deprived of normal lubrication, the eyes become irritated and painful, as if there were something in them. These symptoms are aggravated when the humidity is low or the environment polluted, usually by pollen, dust, or smoke.

When your eyes are chronically dry, you're less comfortable wearing contact lenses, there are fewer tears available when you need to cry, and bright light is hard to take. Early on, these symptoms come and go, but as the dryness continues, the cornea (the transparent membrane that covers the pupil and the iris of the eye) eventually becomes scarred or ulcerated. What started as a few minor symptoms can end up as vision loss.

About 75 percent of people over the age of 65 have some degree of dryness of their eyes. That's because, as we get older, our tear glands make fewer tears and the tears are also less oily.

Age is not the only factor. Pregnant and postmenopausal women are prone to dry eyes, too, presumably because of hormonal changes. And having a faulty immune system can affect the tear glands, proof of which is the fact that one-third of people with rheumatoid arthritis suffer from dry eyes, as do nearly all of the 4 million people nation-wide who have Sjögren's syndrome. Prominent (pop) eyes, caused by an overactive thyroid gland, often become dry because the tears evap-orate too rapidly on the increased surface area.

Whatever is giving you the dry eyes, irrigating them with artificial tears or applying ointments can provide temporary relief, regardless of the underlying problem.

HERE'S WHAT'S NEW

There's good news for the millions of men and women with dry eyes, especially the kind caused by an immune disorder. The FDA has recently approved Restasis, an eyedrop that increases tear production. It is a topical form of cyclosporine, a drug that's otherwise given orally and in much higher doses to suppress the immune system to prevent rejection of transplanted organs. However, tiny amounts, too small to be detected in the blood, are effective when the cyclosporine is used topically as an eyedrop.

In almost 900 patients with dry eye syndrome, Restasis was found to increase tear production by 60 percent so that their vision was less blurred. Their corneas were better lubricated and also had less sur-face damage. The need for artificial tears was reduced by one-third.

Although Restasis was most effective in patients with an auto-immune disorder, it also helped those whose dry eyes were due to "normal" aging.

The drops are taken twice a day; it takes about 3 months for them to work, and they currently cost about $100 a month.

THE BOTTOM LINE

If artificial tears don't relieve your dry eyes, or if you need to take them so often that they interfere with your normal activities, ask your doctor about Restasis eyedrops, especially if you have an autoimmune disorder. This medication is not a cure, but it can significantly improve your symptoms. The drops contain a tiny amount of cyclosporine, a drug that improves the function of the immune system.

Vitamins That Help Macular Degeneration

ADVICE ABOUT VITAMIN SUPPLEMENTS seems to change every day. Remember when vitamin E was a "must" to prevent heart disease? That turned out to be wrong. Vitamin C for colds? This particular debate continues, and I doubt it will ever be resolved, given the passion on both sides of the issue. Beta-carotene (a component of vitamin A) to protect against cancer? Oh boy, were we wrong on that one! Not only does it *not* protect, it actually seems to increase the risk of cancer.

As soon as a vitamin becomes the quick fix for whatever ails you, some researcher finds that it isn't so helpful after all. Regardless, its proponents usually find some other reason to endorse it. Okay, so vitamin E doesn't help the heart, but it *does* reduce the risk of prostate cancer. So there! Too much vitamin D can be toxic, but on the other hand, women need it to keep their bones strong, and both sexes can benefit from its ability to lower their risk of colon cancer.

Despite all these yeas and nays about the potential benefits or detriments of various vitamins, there is universal agreement that anyone over the age of 65 should be taking a multivitamin for general nutritional purposes. That's because many older folks do not predictably eat a balanced diet. This may be because they are bereaved, depressed, alone, or unable to cook for themselves; have poor teeth and can't chew; or simply can't afford a nutritious diet. But whatever the reason, a daily multivitamin helps prevent any significant deficiency. The specific vitamins that the elderly are most likely to lack are the B vitamins, too little of which is a common cause of mental and emotional changes often mistaken for Alzheimer's.

HERE'S WHAT'S NEW

Vitamin supplements slow down macular degeneration, the leading cause of blindness in people older than 60. Macular degeneration is a progressive deterioration of the macula, the central part of the retina responsible for high-resolution vision, such as reading. Someone with macular degeneration can't make out details in their central field of vision. Researchers at Johns Hopkins Medical Institutions in Baltimore have now determined that if every one of the millions of people in this country age 55 and older with early macular degeneration were to take the right vitamin supplements, more than 300,000 of them would avoid more vision loss during the next 5 years.

The original Hopkins study done in 2001 showed that the following vitamin "cocktail," now endorsed in the latest studies, slows the progress of macular degeneration.

- Vitamin C, 500 milligrams

- Vitamin E, 400 IU

- Beta-carotene, 15 milligrams

- Zinc oxide, 80 milligrams

- Cupric oxide (copper), 2 milligrams

The only reservation I have about this multivitamin formula is that anyone who has lung cancer or is at risk for it because of heavy cigarette smoking (past or present) should avoid the beta-carotene. (In smokers, beta-carotene supplements have been associated with an increased risk of lung cancer.)

You can make up this formula yourself by purchasing each item separately, or you can buy the precise formula commercially available as Ocuvite PreserVision and take two tablets twice daily.

Researchers at Brigham and Women's Hospital in Boston were interested in seeing whether the benefit of antioxidant vitamins and carotenoids (compounds responsible for the red, yellow, and orange pigments found in some fruits and vegetables) is also obtained simply by eating enough of these fruits and vegetables themselves. They analyzed the dietary histories of more than 77,000 women and 40,000 men, all of whom were at least 50 years old and whose health status was monitored over a 12- to 18-year period. They found that both sexes who ate 3 or more servings of *fruit* daily had a 36 percent lower risk of age-related macular degeneration compared with those who ate less than 1½ servings a day. Interestingly, the same benefit was apparently not obtained from the vegetables. They also believe that there is greater protection against macular degeneration just from eating fruit often enough rather than taking the vitamin supplements.

THE BOTTOM LINE

Regardless of whether you think you need multivitamin supplements for anything that ails you or threatens your health, it's been proven that the combination of antioxidant vitamins listed above can reduce the rate at which macular degeneration progresses. If you're 55 or older, see your eye doctor for a routine evaluation. If you're told that you either have or are at risk for this common cause of vision loss, start taking these multivitamin supplements now.

Make sure you eat at least 3 servings of fruit a day (the more the better). Some researchers believe that's even better than the vitamins.

How You Sleep Can Affect Your Eyes

IF YOU SNORE AND KEEP YOUR PARTNER AWAKE, and he or she tells you that you suddenly stop breathing for a few seconds many times throughout the night, you almost surely have sleep apnea. Remember, however, that sleep apnea is more than just snoring. The breathing pauses are essential to the diagnosis. This characteristic disturbance of the normal sleep pattern occurs because air cannot flow freely in and out of the nose or mouth, usually as the result of mechanical and structural problems somewhere along the airway. In such cases, breathing is labored and noisy, with frequent short pauses.

Occasionally, sleep apnea occurs because the airways leading to the lungs are obstructed when the throat muscles and the tongue relax during sleep. In obese individuals, excessive tissues may narrow the airways. In another scenario, the uvula (the small fleshy tissue hanging from the center of the back of the throat) loosens up and sags, interfering with the passage of air. Sleep apnea can also be caused by the malfunction of signals from the brain that control breathing.

Whatever the mechanism, sleep apnea almost always results in heavy snoring and frequent, complete cessation of breathing for a few seconds. Drinking alcohol at bedtime or taking sleeping pills increases the frequency and duration of these pauses. The altered breathing often wakes apnea sufferers and abruptly changes their sleep pattern from deep to light.

The most obvious consequence of sleep apnea is chronic fatigue due to lack of sleep. You're exhausted the next day, you don't function efficiently, and you're prone to dozing at the wheel. But sleep apnea is also associated with an increased risk of sudden death, heart attack, stroke, and congestive heart failure—presumably because the lack of oxygen during the breathing pauses adds up. More recently, a higher incidence of gastroesophageal reflux disease (GERD) has been observed in people with sleep apnea.

HERE'S WHAT'S NEW

As if all these problems weren't enough, researchers at the Mayo Clinic in Jacksonville, Florida, report that 33 percent of sleep apnea patients have glaucoma, an important cause of blindness. The incidence of glaucoma in people without sleep apnea is about 2 percent. So sleep apnea is responsible for a 15 times greater risk of developing glaucoma. This complication, like the others, is also probably due to the decreased availability of oxygen that in some way results in increased pressure within the eye. Such elevated intraocular pressure itself causes no symptoms, but if left untreated, can eventually lead to glaucoma and blindness. That's why every adult—especially those with sleep apnea—should have his or her ocular pressure checked at least once a year.

The good news is that sleep apnea can be successfully treated—by removing the airway obstruction (usually surgically); by using continuous positive airway pressure (CPAP), which keeps the airways open with a flow of air through a nasal catheter during the night; or with a dental prosthesis that moves the jaw forward and increases the airflow in the various respiratory passages.

More recently, the FDA approved an effective alternative to CPAP. In this new treatment, known as the Pillar Procedure, a doctor inserts three small woven polyester implants into the roof of the mouth (the soft palate). They are designed to stiffen the soft palate, which collapses to cause airway obstruction in most sleep apnea patients. The procedure itself is minimally invasive, and some patients may find it preferable to CPAP. The cost is between $1,200 and $2,000, about the same as a CPAP device, but much less than surgery.

THE BOTTOM LINE

If you snore and are unusually tired during the day, suspect sleep apnea. If you are found to have it, see an ophthalmologist as well as a sleep specialist. Detection and treatment of elevated ocular pressure can prevent blindness later on. Remember that such elevated pressures do not cause symptoms until it's too late.

There are several effective ways to treat sleep apnea, and the FDA has recently approved a new one.

GALLSTONES

· · · · · · · · · ·

Reduce Your Risk with Coffee

TWENTY MILLION AMERICANS have some problem with their gallbladders—mainly stones, infection, or irritation. Gallstones are usually made up of cholesterol, and symptoms of their presence include
chronic indigestion, nausea, bloating, and excessive burping after
eating a fatty meal. Doctors have traditionally suggested that people
with gallstones avoid coffee. There certainly was no evidence that it
ever prevented them.

HERE'S WHAT'S NEW

First came a study in 1999 from the Harvard School of Public
Health involving 48,000 men followed for 10 years. Those who consumed 2 to 3 cups of coffee every day had a 40 percent lower chance
of having gallstones, while those who drank more than 4 cups a day

had a 45 percent lower risk. This was only true for men who drank caffeinated coffee. Interestingly, caffeinated tea and colas did not have the same protective effect, suggesting that there are constituents in coffee other than caffeine that are responsible for this benefit and that these are obviously not present in decaffeinated coffee.

Then came a 2002 report from the Harvard Nurses' Study, where researchers evaluated the health histories of more than 80,000 nurses between the ages of 34 and 59 years with special attention to their coffee consumption. They found that women who consumed 4 or more cups of caffeinated coffee per day had a 28 percent *lower* risk of developing gallstones than those who did not drink coffee. Drinking 1 to 3 cups a day had a beneficial effect, too, although not quite as much as the higher intake.

THE BOTTOM LINE

Caffeinated coffee protects both men and women from developing gallstones. This is useful information for those of either sex with a family history of such stones.

GOUT

• • • • • • • • • •

Drink Milk to Reduce Gout Attacks

GOUT IS A FORM OF ARTHRITIS that results from excessively high
levels of uric acid in the body, usually the result of eating too much
purine (from excessive alcohol or foods such as red meat, liver,
kidney, brain, or other animal organs that are broken down into uric
acid by the body) or because the kidneys aren't excreting uric acid
normally. Whatever the cause of gout, when there is too much uric
acid in the bloodstream, some is deposited as crystals in one or more
joints, most commonly the big toe, and you wake up one morning
in agony with acute gout. Such attacks recur unpredictably after you
have eaten some dietary no-no or because of unusual stress, or an
infection.

People with chronic excess uric acid in their blood can almost always prevent attacks of gout by taking medications such as Zyloprim (allopurinol), Benemid (probenecid), or colchicine on an ongoing basis. These drugs are usually well-tolerated, but as with any other medication, they can have side effects. Still, if you take them, you can usually remain gout-free and continue to eat what you like, especially if you do so in moderation.

HERE'S WHAT'S NEW

Recent findings will be of interest to anyone who is prone to gout and prefers not to take preventive drugs for whatever reason. In a recent long-term study of more than 47,000 men, several new observations have been made about which foods increase the risk of gout attacks and which protect against them. For example, we used to think that beans, peas, mushrooms, spinach, and cauliflower provoke gout. It turns out that they don't. But an extra portion of beef, pork, or lamb each day does raise the risk of an attack by 21 percent. And just one extra seafood meal a week increases the likelihood by 7 percent, especially (and curiously) in men who are *not* overweight. But drinking between one and five glasses of low-fat milk every day lowers your chances of an acute gout attack by 43 percent! How and why it does so is a mystery, at least to me. Drinking lots of water helps, too, by enabling the kidneys to excrete uric acid from the body.

THE BOTTOM LINE

If you have gout, there are several medications that can drastically lower your risk of an acute attack. Their side effects are usually minimal. If, however, you choose not to use them for any reason and want to rely on diet alone, some new observations will help you reduce the risk of an attack. The most important thing to remember is that drinking between one and five glasses of low-fat milk every day will lower your chances of a gout attack by 43 percent. Drinking lots of water helps, too. Avoid extra portions of meat or seafood and too much booze, especially if you're not taking any of the protective medications.

HEARTBURN

. . . .

Coffee May Go Down Smoothly

CONVENTIONAL WISDOM HAS IT that anyone with heartburn should not drink coffee. You're in for a surprise with this one. Read on.

HERE'S WHAT'S NEW

The effect of coffee on the lower esophageal sphincter, the muscle that separates the upper stomach from the food pipe, varies from person to person, independent of what's going on farther down in the stomach. In other words, it can increase, decrease, or have no effect on the sphincter pressure. In people with heartburn, this pressure tends to be low. The same is true for secretion of acid by the stomach.

Although some studies show that acid production increases after drinking coffee, others do not. So if your heartburn symptoms are aggravated by coffee, either reduce the amount or don't drink it. The same is true for people with stomach ulcers. Coffee can cause or worsen symptoms, but it doesn't do so in everyone. In a recent study of 48,000 men over a 6-year period, there was no association between coffee intake—with or without caffeine—and ulcer formation.

THE BOTTOM LINE

The bad rap coffee has developed over the years in relation to the health of the gastrointestinal tract appears to be unjustified. It may, however, aggravate existing problems in the upper digestive tract (stomach, duodenum, and food pipe) in some people. The only way to determine whether it affects you negatively is to try it. If it worsens your indigestion or ulcer symptoms, then it's no good for you. The point is, if you love coffee and have any of these conditions, don't avoid it simply because of its bad reputation. Try it. Coffee may very well be okay for you.

HEART DISEASE

· · · · · · · · ·

New Relief from Angina

DOCTORS USE THE LATIN TERM *ANGINA PECTORIS* when referring to chest symptoms caused by a specific kind of heart disease in which the coronary arteries become so narrow that not enough blood is available to the heart muscle when it's needed. *Angina* means "pain." *Pectoris* is "chest." The trouble with this term is that the underlying heart problem usually doesn't cause pain; it's more likely to be pressure, heaviness, or simply discomfort, usually behind the breastbone. Nor are these symptoms always limited to the chest. You can experience them in the shoulders, arms, and jaw. Unless you know that angina pectoris does not always mean pain, you may ignore tightness and pressure in the chest and fail to recognize them for what they are—very important warnings on whose proper interpretation your life can depend. Patients whom I subsequently found to have significant heart trouble initially reassured me that they had nothing wrong with their hearts: "no pain, just a heaviness or pressure in the chest."

Angina is the heart's cry for more oxygen. When a coronary artery that supplies the heart is blocked or narrowed by plaques caused by atherosclerosis (hardening of the arteries), it cannot deliver enough blood—and the oxygen it carries—to nourish the cardiac muscles. The offending plaques are composed of fat, calcium, clotted blood, and other substances. As long as the obstruction is only partial, there may be enough blood flow within the artery to satisfy the needs of the heart while you are at rest. So you feel well until you begin to exert yourself or become stressed in any way. At that point the heart needs more blood, the narrowed artery can't deliver it, and you develop angina.

These symptoms are your heart telling you, "Stop what you're doing. I can't handle it." Whether it's tightness, pressure, discomfort, or outright pain, there's something about angina that makes most people instinctively stop what they're doing until the symptoms abate, usually in a minute or two.

To obtain relief virtually immediately, or even to increase the amount of effort you can tolerate before the angina sets in, you can take nitroglycerin, either as a tablet dissolved under the tongue or from a metered oral spray. This medication widens the coronary arteries, allowing more blood to flow through them. If your angina does not respond to nitroglycerin or doesn't clear up when you stop the activity that provoked it, you may be having a heart attack. Therefore, persistent angina is considered a prime emergency that demands immediate professional care.

Angina has such a classic presentation that when you describe your symptoms to your doctor, he or she will usually make the right diagnosis and take steps to confirm it. The typical workup includes a detailed history; a thorough physical exam; blood tests; an electrocardiogram (ECG) taken when you are resting; and if that's normal (which it often is), a stress test (of which there are several different kinds). An exercise test increases the demand for blood by the heart muscle, which if not forthcoming (because the arteries are narrowed) often reproduces your symptoms and results in ECG abnormalities.

Before the days of coronary angiograms, bypass surgery, angioplasty, and stents, we had only medication with which to treat angina. Although drugs are still used in mild cases, if symptoms persist, most cardiologists now recommend that the extent and the severity of the blockages be determined by coronary angiography and removed if necessary, either by angioplasty and stenting, or bypass surgery.

Despite the availability of these newer interventional treatments, it is estimated that more than 6 million men and women in this country have chronic angina because either their arterial blockages are not suitable for surgery or angioplasty or they are among the 26 percent in whom these procedures were not effective.

Patients with ongoing angina need medication to help control their symptoms. Although the effectiveness of these drugs has improved over the years, the relief they provide is limited, and really, no new ones have been approved recently. None can prevent heart attacks and death or provide nearly the same quality of life as successful bypass surgery or angioplasty.

The most important medications for the treatment of chronic angina are mainly long-acting nitroglycerin-type drugs, which widen the narrowed arteries so that they can deliver more blood; beta-blockers, which slow heart rate, lower blood pressure, and reduce the workload on the heart; and various calcium channel blockers, which increase cardiac efficiency.

HERE'S WHAT'S NEW

For the first time in 20 years, an exciting new class of drugs is on the horizon. The prototype is ranolazine (marketed as Ranexa). When taken together with any or all of the currently available medications listed above, it improves angina, especially in patients with weak hearts.

Ranolazine, whose mechanism of action is entirely different from that of any of the other anti-anginal agents, does more than relieve pain. It is a partial fatty acid oxidation (pFOX) inhibitor that causes the heart to use glucose rather than fatty acids for its energy needs. Burning glucose, instead of fatty acids, is more efficient, creates less work for the heart, and reduces its oxygen requirements. As a result, the heart pumps more strongly, permitting you to do more exercise without pain, and there is less need to take nitroglycerin. Ranolazine appears to have few side effects so far, but the FDA was still reviewing the data as this book went to press and has mandated more clinical trials. However, one market analyst predicts the drug will be approved in the second half of 2006. It may be sooner than that if the data continue to be favorable.

THE BOTTOM LINE

If you are one of the more than 6 million Americans with chronic angina, help is on the way. Ranolazine (Ranexa) has been extensively studied and found to increase exercise tolerance safely and effectively when blood supply to the heart is reduced due to coronary artery disease. It works by changing the way in which the heart expends its energy. This drug is still under review by the FDA. I am optimistic, however, based on my interpretation of the data presented so far, that ranolazine will be available in the near future. If you have chronic angina, keep asking your doctor about this medication.

Another Predictor of Heart Trouble

IT HAPPENS ALL THE TIME: Men and women whom you would never suspect to be candidates for heart attacks and strokes suddenly develop them. Their blood pressure, cholesterol, and sugar are all normal; their weight is healthy; they exercise regularly; they've never smoked; they don't drink too much; and their families are long-lived. In short, they're perfect candidates for a long, healthy life. Then one day, out of a clear blue sky, they develop a vascular crisis that neither they nor their doctors expected.

Such attacks happen often enough to have prompted a search for newer, better tests to identify vulnerable individuals who are seemingly not at risk so that doctors can intervene in time. The two most recent and widely used such analyses are of C-reactive protein (C-RP) and homocysteine, elevated levels of which signify increased vulnerability.

HERE'S WHAT'S NEW

A Boston study of more than 3,300 men and women followed through three generations has yielded another measurable protein in the blood that provides a quick and easy way for doctors to predict unexpected heart trouble. It's called B-type natriuretic peptide. As heart muscle begins to weaken, it produces more of this protein to dilate blood vessels and make more oxygen available. This peptide also lowers blood pressure, making it easier for the heart to pump its blood into the arteries.

Measuring the B-type natriuretic peptide level is especially useful in two kinds of situations. The first is in patients who come to the emergency room because they are very short of breath. The clinical exam, chest x-ray, and electrocardiogram may distinguish whether these symptoms are due primarily to a weak heart (congestive heart failure) or to a lung problem (such as emphysema or chronic obstructive lung disease). When the culprit is the heart, the B-type natriuretic peptide level is elevated. Measuring these peptide levels in apparently healthy people is also useful. Those with the highest levels are three times more likely to develop heart failure and 60 percent more likely to die. In addition, twice as many of them are apt to suffer a stroke or develop atrial fibrillation within 5 years.

THE BOTTOM LINE

The best-informed patient gets the best medical care. If in the course of a routine workup your doctor is drawing blood to check your C-RP and homocysteine levels, ask for the B-type natriuretic peptide test, too. The results can help define your vulnerability to vascular disease, regardless of the usual risk factors. Also, if you develop shortness of breath, regardless of whether you think the cause is cardiac or respiratory, quickly go to the nearest emergency room. After you're told the diagnosis, ask the doctor for the results of your B-type natriuretic peptide test. You can be sure he or she will be very impressed.

WHAT THE DOCTOR ORDERED?

COFFEE AND YOUR HEART ● Coffee is probably the most widely consumed, pharmacologically active dietary substance in the United States, where some 160 million people drink it. According to *Consumer Reports* magazine, the average American drinks 3 cups a day. Over the years, there have been many warnings about its dangers, and at least as many kudos about its benefits. For example, research suggests that the regular consumption of coffee reduces the frequency of asthmatic attacks by about 25 percent, and when these attacks do occur, they are apt to be less severe. That's because coffee contains theophylline, a potent dilator of the airways. People with asthma who develop acute wheezing when they don't have their medication with them are urged to drink coffee.

One downside to the regular intake of coffee is the possibility of becoming dependent on it so that if you stop it abruptly, you may experience withdrawal symptoms.

But how does it affect your heart? Traditionally, many doctors believed that coffee wasn't good for the heart. Studies done several years ago reported that strong coffee—either caffeinated or decaffeinated—taken regularly, raises cholesterol levels. In addition, I was taught in medical school (and many doctors are still of the opinion) that moderate coffee consumption, even 2 or 3 cups a day, raises blood pressure. Patients who have any kind of heart rhythm disturbance such as "extra beats" or atrial fibrillation are advised to avoid coffee. Plus, coffee has been reported to significantly raise the blood levels of homocysteine, a protein that is a risk factor for heart disease and stroke.

HERE'S WHAT'S NEW • Whether coffee raises cholesterol levels depends on how the coffee is prepared. According to the latest studies, when ground coffee is boiled or French-press-brewed (as is widely done in Europe), a substance called cafestol is formed—and cafestol does raise cholesterol levels. It takes about 6 cups to produce this effect. But in the United States, where average coffee consumption is 3 cups a day, coffee usually is filtered and percolated, not boiled or French-pressed. Coffee made the American way contains only a trace of cafestol and has not been reported to increase cholesterol levels. Long-term studies on 11,000 Scottish subjects found that the more coffee they drank, the *less* heart disease they had; while coffee consumption by 20,000

Finnish subjects (who drink the "bad" boiled brew) had no effect on the risk of heart disease or death.

With regard to blood pressure, doctors at Johns Hopkins Hospital in Baltimore have found that drinking even 5 cups of coffee a day does not significantly increase blood pressure in healthy men. (Overall, the coffee-drinking men did experience a small increase in blood pressure, but not enough to substantially increase the risk of hypertension.) In those who already have hypertension, however, other studies have shown that eliminating coffee can reduce pressure by as much as 10 points. So if you have hypertension, are in the gray zone, or are under mental stress, it's probably best not to drink coffee.

More recent research from the Medical College of Georgia in Augusta suggests that, at least among adolescents, the association between caffeine intake and systolic pressure (the top figure) varies by race. African American youngsters with the greatest caffeine intake had higher systolic pressure readings than other adolescents. When coffee does raise the pressure, it apparently does so for different reasons in men and women. In females, it increases the force with which the heart contracts, while in men it narrows the blood vessels. Greater consumption probably does increase cardiac irritability.

As far as cardiac arrhythmias are concerned, drinking no more than 3 cups of coffee a day has no effect on heart rhythm, according to the latest studies.

And finally, recent research has confirmed that drinking 6 cups of filtered coffee a day elevates homocysteine levels by about 20 percent. So don't have that much, because raised homocysteine levels can lead to heart disease and stroke. If you must have coffee, take some folic acid, too. (Folid acid supplements lower homocysteine levels.)

THE BOTTOM LINE • Coffee is not bad for your heart and does not raise cholesterol levels, and moderate drinking over a lifetime does not adversely affect your vascular system. But coffee does raise homocysteine levels, so if you're a coffee drinker, take folic acid supplements as well as vitamins B$_6$ and B$_{12}$, which help break down homocysteine in the body.

If your blood pressure is normal, coffee usually will not elevate it. If it is high, however, eliminate coffee for a couple of weeks and see how your pressure responds. If it drops a few points, discuss with your doctor what your coffee limit should be. Adolescent African Americans should limit their coffee intake (and soft drinks that contain caffeine) to 1 cup a day.

Moderate Intake of Alcohol Is Good for You

WE KNOW THAT "some" alcohol is good for you. Teetotalers do not live as long as men and women who imbibe socially, and they also have a higher incidence of heart attack and stroke. That's presumably because alcohol raises the level of "good" HDL, decreases "bad" LDL, lowers blood pressure, reduces the tendency of the blood to clot, increases blood flow within the coronary arteries, and improves the outlook for people with diabetes.

However, in the past, the medical establishment—doctors and their professional associations—and official government bodies have all been wary of actively promoting booze. Instead they have preferred to say that they "tolerate" it. That's because alcohol's benefits to the cardiovascular system (and, more recently, diabetes) are far outweighed by such consequences as violence, drunk driving, and the physical and emotional complications of alcohol addiction. Still, it is important for you to know the pros and cons of drinking in moderation, so that you can act on them as you see fit. Alcohol's benefits should not be hidden because its abuse is dangerous.

HERE'S WHAT'S NEW

After an exhaustive review of the scientific evaluations of alcohol's effects on human health, the U.S. government has made it official. Moderate alcohol consumption is heart healthy. It has also defined "moderate alcohol consumption" as no more than one drink per day for women and two drinks for men. Beer and wine offer the same protection against cardiovascular disease, including heart attack and stroke. These conclusions were included in a new set of guidelines issued by the government in 2004.

Doctors at the National Institute of Alcohol Abuse and Alcoholism emphasize that these recommendations are not for pregnant women, women with a family history of breast cancer, or those on estrogen replacement therapy. Nor do they apply to anyone who operates a vehicle, is an alcoholic, or has a family history of alcoholism.

This government position is not meant to encourage anyone who is not a drinker to start now. But if you do enjoy alcohol in moderation, and are able to handle it, you should know that it is actually good for you.

THE BOTTOM LINE

If you enjoy a glass or two of wine or a cocktail at dinner, you will surely welcome this official recommendation. Remember, however, that although a couple of drinks a day are good for you, more is not better. Stay within these guidelines, and you'll remain healthy; exceed them, and you're looking for trouble.

Does Aspirin Help a Healthy Heart?

AN ASPIRIN A DAY definitely reduces the risk of having a *second* heart attack or stroke. Some studies have suggested that it can also prevent a first attack.

HERE'S WHAT'S NEW

If you've had any doubts about the benefit of taking aspirin while you're still healthy, a new analysis using data from the Physicians' Health Study should convince you of the wisdom of doing so. Researchers at Yale University analyzed the results from five studies in which aspirin was given to more than 55,000 healthy people, more than 11,000 of whom were women. They found that the drug reduced the risk of a first heart attack by 32 percent and lowered the incidence of all major cardiac events by 15 percent during the next 10 years.

On the basis of these findings, they recommend that you assess your risk of having a first heart attack based on a number of factors. These include age (the older you are, the more vulnerable you are), gender (premenopausal women are not normally at high risk and would not need such protection), weight (overweight is an important risk factor), family history (genes play a role), diabetes (a very important threat that requires all the protection you can get against vascular disease, including prophylactic aspirin), smoking (another very big danger), and high blood cholesterol and blood pressure levels (again, major risk factors).

These researchers believe that aspirin is currently not used often enough to prevent first heart attacks. It is estimated that if more people took aspirin, 150,000 cardiovascular deaths could be prevented each year. Although aspirin can cause gastrointestinal bleeding, especially in the elderly, and also carries with it a small chance of a hemorrhagic stroke, particularly in someone with high blood pressure, these dangers are not nearly as great as the likelihood of heart attack or stroke without preventive aspirin.

The researchers also recommend that patients with a high-risk profile for heart attack should also take a cholesterol-lowering drug (statin), regardless of their cholesterol levels. Furthermore, it goes without saying that exercising, eliminating tobacco, and controlling weight and high blood pressure are very important, too.

The recommended maintenance dose of preventive aspirin is an 81-milligram tablet, preferably uncoated, taken each day.

THE BOTTOM LINE

Although aspirin is now widely used to prevent a second heart attack or stroke, it can also help avoid one in otherwise healthy people with such risk factors as high cholesterol levels, elevated blood pressure, cigarette smoking, overweight, a family history of heart disease, and diabetes.

WHAT THE DOCTOR ORDERED?

DHEA—HYPE AND HOPE • In the 2004 edition of *Breakthrough Health,* I reported that DHEA had not been found to help patients with Alzheimer's disease. To refresh your memory, DHEA (dehydroepiandrosterone) is produced by the adrenal glands and later converted mainly into estrogen and progesterone. This "wonder" drug remains a huge seller in health food stores and on the Internet. The rationale for its use is the fact that when we're young, we have high levels of DHEA in the blood, and as we age, we have progressively less. Those who advocate its use believe that replenishing DHEA will slow the aging process.

HERE'S WHAT'S NEW • Research on DHEA continues in animals and humans. Some new studies suggest that it may help prevent heart attacks. For example, researchers at the Kumamoto University School of Medicine in Japan reported in the *Journal of Clinical Endocrinology and Metabolism* that 25 milligrams per day of DHEA in men with elevated cholesterol resulted in significant improvement in the lining of the coronary arteries, as well as increased sensitivity to insulin (factors that increase coronary blood flow). DHEA was also found to benefit some patients with mild to moderate lupus, an autoimmune disorder that affects many organs. Lupus patients taking DHEA sometimes required lower doses of steroids to control their symptoms.

According to French scientist Etienne-Emile Beaulieu, a pioneer in DHEA research, this supplement can reduce abnormally elevated pressure in the lungs of rats. Chronic hypoxic pulmonary hypertension is a serious and widespread disorder in humans that is extremely difficult to treat. If Beaulieu's observations on the effect of DHEA in rats can be shown to apply to humans, it will be of enormous and practical importance.

But here's the other side of the coin. In a paper published in the *Journal of the American College of Cardiology,* researchers at the Royal Prince Albert Hospital in Sydney, Australia, concluded that DHEA causes certain blood cells to suck up cholesterol. These "foam cells," as they're called when they do so, then form plaques within the coronary arteries. When these plaques rupture, they can obstruct the artery and cause a heart attack.

Earlier studies reported in last year's edition of *Breakthrough Health* that found no effect from DHEA on patients with Alzheimer's disease were reinforced by subsequent observations from the University of California, San Francisco. Researchers there reported that Alzheimer's patients taking DHEA for 6 months showed no significant difference in performance, severity of the disease, or the rate of its progression.

THE BOTTOM LINE • Here's the DHEA scorecard at the present time:

• Evidence of its effectiveness for heart disease is conflicting.

• Some patients with lupus may benefit and require lower doses of steroids to control their disease.

• Patients with Alzheimer's disease do not respond to this therapy.

The potential downside from the use of DHEA continues to be relevant.

While it is possible that in the future DHEA may prove to be beneficial, I still do not recommend it to my patients. If, however, you're looking for a "quick fix" toward immortality and are willing to accept the possible risks associated with this supplement, ask your doctor to prescribe it but to do so from a pharmacy where you're more likely to get a standardized product.

Remember that the FDA does not oversee the production of any supplements. In a recent analysis of several DHEA products sold in health food stores and over the Internet, the bottles did not always contain what the label claimed was present; some had much less, others much more. One preparation was even made from the adrenal glands of cows, raising at least a theoretical risk (however remote) of contracting mad cow disease. I'd much rather get sick from steak.

Surprising News about Homocysteine

IN THE 2004 EDITION of *Breakthrough Health,* I wrote the following: "Homocysteine is a protein by-product of normal metabolism. Its levels can be measured in the blood. When they're too high, you're at increased risk for heart attack, high blood pressure, stroke, and blood clots in the deep veins of the leg. . . . If your homocysteine level is high, each day you should take 1 milligram of folic acid (the supplemental form of folate), as well as 10 milligrams of vitamin B_6 and 400 micrograms of vitamin B_{12}. *The hard proof that lowering homocysteine actually prevents heart attacks is not yet in, but most researchers are confident that it will do so."*

HERE'S WHAT'S NEW

Well, guess what? Most researchers may have been wrong! According to a large study at Wake Forest University School of Medicine in Winston-Salem, North Carolina, published in the *Journal of the American Medical Association,* 1,840 patients with a previous stroke and elevated homocysteine levels who were given high-dose vitamin therapy did *not* have a lower incidence of stroke, heart disease, and death in the following 2 years—even though this therapy did reduce their homocysteine levels. Patients in a control group given only a token dose of this vitamin combination and in whom the homocysteine levels did not drop had the same incidence of subsequent vascular events than the treated group.

The other important news about homocysteine is that it appears to be more than just a marker of increased risk for heart attack and stroke. High levels of this protein in both men and women also reflect an increased risk for developing osteoporosis—the higher the level, the greater the chance that the bones will become thin and break easily. Whether or not normalizing homocysteine levels will affect the risk of osteoporosis is still not clear. If, however, your homocysteine level is high, you should, in addition to taking folic acid supplements, do whatever is necessary to preserve the health of your bones: exercise regularly; consume enough calcium, either in the diet or in supplements; and when necessary, take one or more of the anti-osteoporosis drugs now on the market.

Another recent (and, again, unexpected) observation relates to the effect of folic acid in men with high homocysteine levels who undergo angioplasty and receive bare-metal stents. Surprisingly, there is a *greater* chance that these stents will close. (This does not apply to women, people with diabetes, or those whose homocysteine levels are essentially normal.)

THE BOTTOM LINE

Several of my patients for whom I had prescribed folic acid to lower their homocysteine levels adopted the attitude that this was a quick fix for their problems, that it would prevent any vascular problems, and that they could continue to gain weight, be couch potatoes, smoke—and generally lead unhealthy lives. But recent data indicate that lowering the homocysteine level with the appropriate trio of B vitamins apparently does not reduce the risks associated with these abnormal concentrations, and that one must also vigorously continue to control every other risk factor that contributes to stroke and heart attack.

It may very well be that homocysteine is only a marker or predictor of vascular disease and that lowering it makes no difference. However, there may be other interpretations of these unexpected study results. Remember that the subjects in this study had already suffered a heart attack or stroke. Perhaps the vitamin B treatment should be started *before* the vascular disease has occurred. These vitamins may not do any good *after* the damage has been done. The other possibility is that it may take longer than 2 years for these vitamins to work and that the study might have shown different results years later.

The observation that lowering an elevated homocysteine level is associated with a greater chance that bare-metal stents inserted after angioplasty will close up is very disturbing. If you are scheduled for such a stent procedure, discuss this recent news with your doctor. He or she may decide that you should stop folate therapy prior to the revascularization procedure.

Here's my advice: If you have an elevated homocysteine level, take folic acid, B_6, and B_{12} vitamins in the doses suggested above. They can do no harm, and they may possibly help prevent vascular disease years later and decrease your vulnerability to osteoporosis. However, do not take them if you are about to have angioplasty and bare-metal stenting.

WHAT THE DOCTOR ORDERED?

EATING FISH FENDS OFF SUDDEN DEATH • During the last few years, doctors have become convinced that eating cold-water fish—especially fatty ones such as herring, sardines, salmon, and tuna—protects against heart disease, high blood pressure, arthritis, ulcerative colitis, some cancers, and much of whatever ails mankind. It also improves mental health. Eskimos and other populations consuming the largest amount of such seafood generally have a lower incidence of these diseases.

The constituents in fish that confer this protection are the omega-3 group of essential fatty acids, notably eicosapentaenoic acid (EPA) and docosahexanoic acid (DHA), present exclusively in these marine animals. Although alpha-linolenic acid (ALA) found in flaxseed and flaxseed oil is also an omega-3 fatty acid, very little of it is actually converted to EPA and DHA, and so taking ALA supplements is not a substitute for eating fish. The recommended amounts of these cold-water fish are at least two servings a week, or about 2 grams of omega-3 capsules a day. Fish oils, no matter how you take them, also possess anticlotting properties. If you take them along with an anticoagulant drug, such as Coumadin (warfarin), which "thins" the blood, have your blood clotting monitored regularly.

HERE'S WHAT'S NEW • An interesting study in the *Lancet* suggests even more benefits from fish oils. It seems that EPA and DHA can prevent sudden cardiac death. This was determined in an ingenious experiment carried out by German researchers who evaluated 10 people previously determined to be especially vulnerable to sudden cardiac death. They all had received an implanted defibrillator that would shock the heart back to normal rhythm whenever such a threatening rhythm developed.

The researchers then tried to trigger this life-threatening arrhythmia in these patients (who were protected by their implanted defibrillators). They found this was more difficult to do in those patients who had been given an infusion of fish oils.

The findings in this small experiment confirm earlier observations by Italian researchers in 2002. A group of 11,300 participants were divided into four groups who received either 1 gram daily of omega-3 fatty acids or a variety of placebos. There were significantly fewer sudden deaths among those who took the supplements.

This important cardioprotective property is not limited to the fish oil extracts or capsules. Researchers at the Brigham and Women's Hospital and Harvard Medical School, both in Boston, recently reported that the regular intake of baked or broiled (but not fried) fish reduced the risk of atrial fibrillation (a potentially serious cardiac rhythm abnormality that affects 2 million Americans). Among almost 5,000 people over the age of 65 whom they assessed twice— at the beginning and the end of an 11-year span—there were 980 cases of atrial fibrillation. Those who reported eating baked or broiled fish such as tuna one to four times a week had a 28 percent lower risk of developing this arrhythmia than those who ate it less than once a month.

THE BOTTOM LINE • I advise my patients who are at risk for heart disease, or who already have it, either to eat plenty of fish or take omega-3 capsule supplements, especially if they have a cardiac rhythm disorder.

Vitamins—To E or Not to E

ONE OF THE REASONS that I enjoy writing these updates so much is that I get to share with my readers how so many medical facts become medical myths. Vitamin E is an excellent example. A report in the *Nutrition Reporter* newsletter in 1995 summed up the existing and accepted state of our knowledge at the time. The piece starts by saying, "The 50-year-old controversy surrounding the role of vitamin E in preventing coronary heart disease came to an end of sorts 2 years ago. That's when Harvard University researchers reported that supplemental doses of the vitamin reduce the risk of heart disease by as much as 54 percent."

At the time, this was an accurate assessment of all the research available relating to the role of vitamin E in the prevention and management of heart disease. It summed up the results of many studies here and abroad, most of which have since been proven flawed in one way or another—too few study participants, limited duration of treatment, and the inability to distinguish if the beneficial results were due to the vitamin E or other lifestyle factors. Virtually every doctor who was keeping up with the literature at the time recommended vitamin E supplements to his or her patients who either had coronary artery disease or were vulnerable to it. Note that I use the word *supplements*, because there has never been any doubt that a diet rich in antioxidant-containing foods (fruits, vegetables, and whole grains) does reduce disease of the heart and blood vessels.

HERE'S WHAT'S NEW

Researchers at McMaster University in Hamilton, Ontario, conducted a randomized, double-blind, placebo-controlled trial, testing whether vitamin E reduces the risk of heart attack, stroke, or cardiovascular death in more than 9,500 high-risk patients. After 7 years, they found that 15.2 percent of those taking vitamin E had a heart attack, compared with 14.3 percent of those on placebo; 5.7 percent of the vitamin E patients had a stroke, compared with 5.1 percent of those on placebo; just over 10 percent of those on vitamin E died from cardiovascular causes, compared with 9.9 percent of those on placebo. These results confirm another study, carried out in the United States and published in the journal *Circulation*, that found vitamin E to have no preventive effect on heart attack in men who took it over a 13-year period.

The McMaster University team also evaluated the effects of vitamin E on cancer and again found no statistical differences compared with a placebo. On the contrary, there was a statistically significant 17 percent *increase* in the risk of congestive heart failure in those taking the vitamin. These findings should end the love affair between vitamin E and arteriosclerosis that has impassioned so many of us for so long.

Nonetheless, we should not abandon research into vitamin E's possible benefits in other areas such as macular degeneration, prostate cancer, and Alzheimer's. There is evidence that it may play a role in treating these diseases. Also, recent published work indicates that vitamin E supplements reduce the incidence of the common cold (but not more serious respiratory ailments such as the flu) in the elderly.

THE BOTTOM LINE

Impressive and definitive studies on the role of vitamin E *supplements* in preventing or modifying existing heart disease indicate that they are of no benefit in this area. However, foods rich in this vitamin do appear to be protective. This does not apply to the possible benefit of vitamin E supplements in other disorders.

WHAT THE DOCTOR ORDERED?

CHECKUP OR CHECK OUT • A regular checkup with your doctor used to be as American as apple pie. These days, however, the "cost-effectiveness" experts among us are questioning whether it's worth it. For example, they point out that it takes many thousands of dollars to do enough routine colonoscopies on people without symptoms just to find one silent cancer early enough to cure. In their view, that's not cost efficient. Of course, it depends on whose life is saved. If it was their lives, I assure you they would consider the money well spent.

Despite the economic and political wrangling surrounding routine screening, it's my impression that most men and women still want to be seen by their doctors on a regular basis to detect the earliest evidence of diseases to which they are particularly vulnerable by virtue of their age, family history, gender, race, occupation, and other personal characteristics. But most healthy people are never sure when to start such screening and how often to have it done.

HERE'S WHAT'S NEW • In a historic move, the American Cancer Society, the American Diabetes Association, and the American Heart Association have agreed upon and published screening guidelines to reduce the risk of cancer, diabetes, heart disease, and stroke—four diseases that account for nearly two of every three deaths annually in the United States. In addition, they have emphasized four basic health messages.

• Eat a healthy diet to maintain optimal weight.

• Exercise regularly, ideally 30 minutes a day, 5 days a week.

• Avoid smoking and exposure to secondhand smoke.

• Visit a doctor regularly to assess your personal health risks.

Here is a checklist for the screenings and tests these organizations recommend for the general adult population. Photocopy it, post it on your fridge, and take it with you to the doctor at every checkup.

❏ Blood pressure. Get it measured every 2 years starting at age 20. (I also suggest that children in families where high blood pressure is common should have their readings taken starting at age 3.)

❏ Body mass index (BMI). Have it calculated at every regular checkup starting at age 20. (You should discuss the frequency of these routine physicals with your doctor.) Many doctors prefer the BMI measurement for evaluating optimal weight. You can figure out yours by using the following mathematical formula: Your BMI equals your weight (in kilograms) divided by your height (in square meters). For both men and women, the normal range for BMI is between 20 and 24.9. You are overweight if your BMI is between 25 and 29; a BMI over 30 means you are obese.

❏ Cholesterol (and its components such as HDL and LDL). Get it checked every 5 years starting at age 20.

❏ Blood glucose. Have it tested every 3 years starting at age 45.

❏ Colorectal screening. Depending on the test used, have this done starting at age 50. Several tests detect colorectal cancer, including an annual examination of the stool for the presence of blood; a sigmoidoscopy (in which only the lower portion of the bowel is examined); and a colonoscopy, which views the entire length of the colon. Unless there is a strong family history of cancer or the test indicates the presence of polyps, a sigmoid-oscopy is done every 5 years, and a colonoscopy, every 10 years.

❑ Clinical breast exam (for women). Have one every 3 years starting at age 20, yearly after age 40. (Breast self-exams are no longer officially recommended, but I suggest you do them when-ever you can and have an annual mammogram after age 40.)

❑ Pap test (for women). Go for this test annually starting at age 20, and every 1 to 3 years after age 30.

❑ Prostate specific antigen, or PSA test (for men). This testing is controversial, so discuss it with your doctor. I have it done on every male patient over the age of 50, and sometimes younger. And you should discuss with your doctor having a digital rectal exam if you are age 50 or older (see page 65).

THE BOTTOM LINE • You no longer have any excuse for not complying with the steps needed to keep yourself healthy and to detect and prevent diseases that can cripple and kill you. Do it ex-actly as these three great medical associations recommend—you won't regret it.

New Treatment Guidelines for Women

THE INCIDENCE OF HEART DISEASE in premenopausal women is very low. But come menopause, cardiac problems kick in with a vengeance and become the leading cause of death in females, killing nearly half a million of them each year in this country alone—one every minute.

The total mortality from heart disease and stroke in women is greater than the next seven causes of death combined—including all forms of cancer. Still, because the medical profession and women themselves have been so inculcated with the notion that heart trouble is a male problem, they have paid little attention to this reality. Most women still mistakenly view breast cancer as the greatest threat to their survival.

HERE'S WHAT'S NEW

The U.S. government and the American Heart Association (AHA) have now officially recognized the threat to women from cardiovascular disease. Whereas the focus used to be on the management of *existing* heart disease, the emphasis now is on recognizing the presence of risk factors and stressing the importance of their modification *before* menopause.

This new position is also different and important because it concentrates on an individual woman's cardiovascular health status rather than on the gender as a whole. The former recommendations were based on "does she or does she not have a heart condition?" The new ones take into consideration the fact that women are *vulnerable* to heart disease for all kinds of reasons and that no single management regimen fits all.

Several risk categories have been established, the most important of which are high, intermediate, and optimal. Here is how each is defined and the intervention recommended by the AHA for each category.

High. This risk category includes any woman at any age who already has definite evidence of vascular disease, such as coronary artery disease (usually manifested as angina or a previous heart attack) or arterial disease anywhere else in the body—for example, the legs, the kidneys, or the carotid artery in the neck. Diabetes is also included because it is so often associated with vascular disease. (More than 70 percent of diabetic men and women ultimately develop some kind of vascular problem, and at least 65 percent of people with diabetes die from heart disease or stroke.)

Intermediate. Women with multiple risk factors without evidence of frank disease fall into this category. These risk factors include one or more of the following: high blood pressure, abnormal cholesterol, overweight, tobacco use, and pre-diabetes (higher-than-normal blood sugar, but not so high as to qualify as diabetes). Obviously, the urgency of intervention depends on the severity of risk factors and how many there are. A woman's genetic history is also important in this category. If any of her first-degree relatives—mother, father, brother, or sister—had cardiovascular disease, such as a heart attack, relatively early in life (before 55 years of age in the men or younger than 65 in women), she belongs in the intermediate risk category.

Optimal. The optimal level includes women without any significant risk factors who follow a heart-healthy lifestyle described below.

How to prevent or treat your personal risk factors depends on the category into which you fall. However, there are certain guidelines that apply to all women. For example, women should avoid smoking and reduce their exposure to secondhand smoke as much as possible. It's not enough to quit smoking—immediate family members need to give it up, too. Those who insist on lighting up, should do so outside, just as they would in restaurants, hospitals, office buildings, and other public places. Whether a wife chooses to invoke any other means of persuading her husband to quit is, of course, up to her. But I can tell you from experience, persuasion does work. I quit (under duress) 45 years ago.

Exercise is probably one of the most important ways to reduce the risk of vascular disease. Every woman should perform at least 30 minutes of moderate-intensity physical activity such as brisk walking, preferably every day. You can exercise at home on a treadmill or outdoors, depending on the weather. The key, however, is to do the kind of exercise you enjoy. High-risk women who've had a heart attack, angina, angioplasty, or a bypass operation should enroll in a comprehensive risk-reduction regimen that includes cardiac rehabilitation. There are many such programs throughout the country, often at local hospitals.

A heart-healthy diet is also universally recommended, and in the opinion of the AHA, that does not mean a low-carbohydrate, high-saturated-fat regimen such as the Atkins diet. An overall healthy eating pattern should include a variety of fruits, vegetables, grains, low-fat or fat-free dairy products, legumes, and plenty of fish and other sources of protein low in saturated fat. The best protein-rich foods are poultry and other lean meats, fish, rice, beans, and wheat germ. Total fat intake should be less than 10 percent of the total calories consumed, but in high-risk women, less than 7 percent is recommended.

Weight control is another lifestyle recommendation. Do whatever is necessary, and I don't mean liposuction (see page 209), to maintain a waist circumference of less than 35 inches and a body mass index below 25 (see page 142).

High-risk women who are depressed should be treated so that they will remain motivated to follow the proper lifestyle or control their risk factors.

They are also advised to take omega-3 fatty acid supplements of oily, cold-water fish such as tuna, salmon, and herring. The DHA and EPA they contain have recently been shown to protect against sudden cardiac death (see page 137) and various forms of cancer, including breast cancer. I am puzzled as to why *all* women are not advised to take these supplements.

Homocysteine is a protein in the blood that when elevated is a marker for heart attack and stroke (see page 134). In such cases, a doctor may prescribe folic acid, often along with vitamins B_6 and B_{12}. In the new guidelines, folic acid is recommended for high-risk women with increased homocysteine levels. In my view, all women should take folic acid, not only those at high risk.

Here is how the AHA suggests dealing with major risk factors.

Control your blood pressure. That's extremely important in every category. You can do it effectively only if you're checked often enough to detect it. No matter what kind of doctor you see, whether it's a dermatologist or gynecologist, insist on having your blood pressure taken at every visit. Your goal should be a reading of 120/80. The first step is a low-salt diet (particularly important for African Americans who are especially sensitive to excessive salt), weight control, and exercise.

Many people develop high blood pressure despite a healthy lifestyle. If your reading is greater than 140/90, or even somewhat lower than that and you also have diabetes, you will probably need medication. In the old days, virtually all of the blood-pressure-lowering drugs had intolerable side effects. Today, many of them normalize pressure effectively without toxicity, so there's no excuse for anyone to have high blood pressure. Make sure, however, whatever combination of drugs you're taking and regardless of your risk category, that one of them is a thiazide (a water pill or diuretic). High-risk women, especially if they have any heart failure, should also take an angiotensin converting enzyme (ACE) inhibitor such as Capoten (captopril), Prinivil or Zestril (lisinopril), or Altace (ramipril). These drugs strengthen the heart muscle. Unfortunately, ACE inhibitors can cause a dry, irritating cough. If you happen to develop one, take an angiotensin receptor blocker (ARB) drug instead, such as Cozaar (losartan), Avapro (irbesartan), Diovan (valsartan), Benicar (olmesartan), or one of the many others available. They act virtually the same way as the ACE inhibitors but usually do not cause a cough.

Lower your cholesterol levels. Normalizing your cholesterol level is extremely important. Optimal numbers for men and women are an LDL (bad cholesterol) less than 100, although newer research indicates that it should be closer to 60 or 70 for anyone who already has heart trouble. HDL (good cholesterol) should be greater than 50. Triglycerides—which are measured after you've been fasting overnight—should be under 150. Total cholesterol minus the HDL should be below 130.

The AHA recommends different treatment approaches for abnormal cholesterol in each of the risk groups. I disagree with this position because I believe that everyone whose cholesterol profile is abnormal should be treated with equal vigor. Here, for the record, are the AHA guidelines.

Everyone should first try diet. In my own experience, this alone is rarely enough over the long term. Most of my patients end up needing medication, too. According to the AHA, high-risk women whose cholesterol is greater than 200 should reduce their saturated-fat intake to less than 7 percent of total calories consumed and eat as few foods containing trans fatty acids as possible. (These are present in foods such as commercial cookies, crackers, french fries, microwave popcorn, vegetable shortening, and some margarines—indeed any packaged food that lists "partially hydrogenated vegetable oil" or "shortening" among its ingredients.) These trans fatty acids raise the LDL, lower the HDL, and may also lead to type 2 diabetes.

In high-risk women, the drugs of choice when the LDL is greater than 100 are the statins, such as Lipitor (atorvastatin), Zocor (simvastatin), and others. When the HDL is low, niacin or fibrate therapy is recommended instead of the statin.

I believe everyone with an abnormal lipid (blood fat) profile should take these steps. However, according to the AHA, in the intermediate group, statins should be started only when the LDL is greater than or equal to 130. Among the lower risk groups, the AHA recommends deferring treatment until the LDL is 190 or greater! I hope and expect that these guidelines will be changed. I know of no doctor who would follow them.

Try to achieve near-normal blood sugar levels if you are diabetic. That's your best guarantee of avoiding the vascular complications of this disease. Also, check your own blood sugar regularly and have what is called a hemoglobin A1c (HgA1c) test every few weeks. This tells you what your blood sugar average has been over the past few days (the reading should be less than 6 percent). This test is more informative than a single blood sugar determination. Previously, your doctor had to determine the HgA1c, but in the last few months a machine has become available that allows you to do it yourself.

The latest twist on the HgA1c test is that it's more than an indicator of adequate sugar control. It *also* predicts the risk of developing heart disease in non-diabetics. People with HgA1c concentrations of less than 5 percent have the lowest rates of cardiovascular disease and mortality. Some doctors believe that this test should be added to the list of other clearly established risk factors for heart disease, such as blood pressure and cholesterol. Weight loss by means of diet and exercise, as well as sugar-lowering drugs, insulin, or both, may be necessary to achieve optimal blood sugar levels.

Stabilize heart rhythm disorders. There is a common chronic heart rhythm disorder called atrial fibrillation. It can occur in otherwise normal people, but it is usually a manifestation of some underlying heart disease, especially a valve disorder. People with this arrhythmia should have their blood "thinned" in order to prevent a stroke. The drug of choice here is Coumadin (warfarin). However, in anyone at risk for internal bleeding from Coumadin, aspirin is considered to be safe.

But what about aspirin for people with normal rhythm? You should certainly take it if you're in the high and intermediate risk groups for vascular disease but not if you're risk-free. The latest information is that uncoated aspirin tablets may be more protective than the coated ones. But remember that aspirin can irritate the intestinal tract and cause bleeding. Older people who take it on a regular basis should have their stool checked for the presence of blood. You can't always see that blood, and it has to be detected chemically with stool-analysis cards that you can either buy at a drugstore or obtain from your doctor. Women at high risk who cannot tolerate aspirin should take Plavix (clopidogrel), which also has anticlotting properties.

If you've had any previous heart trouble, you should also take a beta-blocker, such as Tenormin (atenolol), Inderal (propranolol), or Coreg (carvedilol), in addition to aspirin, but not if you have chronic lung disease. Discuss this one with your doctor. ACE inhibitors such as Altace (ramipril) or Vasotec (enalapril) are also frequently prescribed.

Consider hormone therapy. I think everyone now knows that estrogen alone or combined with progesterone should not be used routinely by postmenopausal women. Similarly, the AHA guidelines do not recommend that these hormones be taken to prevent cardiovascular disease. However, I personally think that some women have overreacted to this recommendation. If you are suffering from menopausal symptoms such as severe hot flashes, take the hormones in the smallest effective dose for the shortest period of time. The complications from the long-term use of these hormones, though real, are relatively uncommon.

Avoid antioxidant supplements. One thing that may surprise you is the official position on antioxidant vitamins such as E and C, which are now suspected of actually aggravating heart disease. They also appear to interfere with the action of the cholesterol-lowering statin drugs. I have stopped recommending them to my patients and anyone taking a statin. Instead of these supplements, eat plenty of the foods that contain these vitamins, such as fruits and leafy green vegetables. Remember that removing a vitamin or any other ingredient of a natural food and putting it into a pill does not have the same effect as eating that food.

THE BOTTOM LINE

The medical profession is finally paying attention to the vascular problems of women. In the past, we acted as if only men were vulnerable to them. This new focus is the result of the realization that heart disease kills more women than the next seven leading causes of death combined—including cancer. In this country one woman dies every minute from heart disease. Although such vascular disease occurs after menopause, risk factors are present early in life. They should be looked for and treated. Appropriate lifestyle changes can reduce its incidence if started early enough.

WHAT THE DOCTOR ORDERED?

THE PROS AND CONS OF A VEGETARIAN DIET

There are several different kinds of vegetarians, all of whom avoid eating meat. The major types are *vegans,* who exclude eggs, dairy, and all other animal products; *lacto-ovo vegetarians,* who eat mainly grains, vegetables, fruits, legumes, seeds, nuts, dairy products, and eggs, and avoid meat, fish, and poultry; *lacto-vegetarians,* who eat everything but animal flesh and eggs; *ovo-vegetarians,* who eschew animal flesh and dairy products but eat eggs; *semi-vegetarians,* who abstain only from red meat; and *pesco-vegetarians,* who eat fish, dairy, and eggs but no meat or poultry.

People have different reasons for following a meat-free diet. Some do so because eating animal products is against their religion, or they believe it violates animal rights or it is simply healthier. Others just don't like the taste of meat. Whatever the reason, are these vegetarian diets healthier than those containing meat? For people with certain medical problems, such as kidney failure, a vegetarian-based diet may be absolutely necessary. On the other hand, someone at risk for developing ovarian or testicular cancer should avoid strict vegan diets that contain high levels of potassium and zinc.

Most doctors have no problem with their patients being vegetarian, as long as certain precautions discussed below are taken. I do not believe that vegetarians are any healthier than those who eat a well-balanced diet of nutritious foods that are fresh and unprocessed. However, according to the American Dietetic Association, an appropriately planned vegetarian diet is healthy and nutritionally adequate, and it reduces the risk of obesity, osteoporosis, and cancer. There is also suggestive evidence that such a diet lowers the likelihood of high blood pressure, coronary artery disease, type 2 diabetes, and gallstones.

Do nonmeat eaters live longer? According to statistics, the life span of vegetarians is about the same or maybe slightly longer than that of nonvegetarians, but any increase, at least in this country, may be due to nondietary lifestyle factors to which vegetarians seem to adhere more closely than meat eaters—refraining from smoking, abstaining from alcohol or using it only moderately, being physically active, getting enough rest, and seeing the doctor when necessary.

What about cancer? The National Cancer Institute states that one-third of cancer deaths are related to diet. Vegetables from the cabbage family (cruciferous) as well as diets low in saturated fat and high in fiber may reduce the risk of certain types of malignancies. The lower incidence of type 2 diabetes in these individuals is the result of a higher intake of complex carbohydrates and a lower body mass index.

The downside to the vegetarian diets is that the stricter they are, the more difficult it is to get all the necessary nutrients. Vegetarians who exclude all dairy and animal flesh products are especially at risk because some essential nutrients exist only in animal products. Vegans may have inadequate vitamin and mineral levels; the most important is B_{12}, a deficiency of which can lead to irreversible nerve damage. That's why I don't believe that elderly people, whose absorption of dietary B_{12} from the stomach is reduced anyway, should adopt a vegetarian diet. Vegetarians who avoid dairy products may also consume too little vitamin D and calcium, which predisposes them to osteoporosis. These vegetarians are also at risk for iron deficiency, an important cause of anemia, not only because they don't eat animal products but also because excess fiber in their diets inhibits the absorption of iron from the stomach and leads to anemia. They may also be protein deficient and lose hair and muscle mass.

Vegetarian diets pose additional risks and health concerns for children. Lack of vitamin D causes rickets. They may lack the dietary iron they would get from consuming animal products and the equally valuable copper and zinc. Copper is essential for normal function of the immune system and strengthens red blood cells. Protein deficiency stunts a child's growth. Women of childbearing age who follow a vegetarian diet have a greater chance of having irregular periods, and when they do become pregnant, they may deliver babies with low birth weight.

HERE'S WHAT'S NEW • New research now suggests that even those vegetarians who are more lenient in their diets are also at risk for vitamin B_{12} deficiency. German researchers reporting in the *American Journal of Clinical Nutrition* evaluated 174 apparently healthy people living in Germany and the Netherlands. They found that 92 percent of the vegans they studied—that is, those who ate the strictest vegetarian diet, which shuns all animal products, including milk and eggs—were vitamin B_{12} deficient. Also 77 percent of people who followed a vegetarian diet that included milk and eggs as their only food of animal origin also had too little B_{12}. On the other hand, only 11 percent of those who ate meat had vitamin B_{12} deficiency that can not only cause nerve damage but also elevate blood levels of homocysteine, an amino acid implicated as a marker for increased risk of heart disease and stroke (see page 134). Unlike some other B vitamins, B_{12} is not present in any plant food other than fortified cereals, but it is plentiful in meat and fish. Milk and eggs contain smaller amounts.

Even young, healthy meat-eaters may not be getting enough B_{12}. One study found that nearly 40 percent of 3,000 adults ages 26 to 83 had blood levels of vitamin B_{12} low enough to cause problems. This is likely due to the increased use of antacids that block the absorption of vitamin B_{12} from the stomach.

No adverse effects have ever been associated with an excess of B_{12} from food or supplements in healthy individuals. You can't have too much of it.

THE BOTTOM LINE • Vegetarians, anyone taking antacids on an ongoing basis, and seniors should take oral vitamin B_{12} supplements in a dose of 0.5 to 1 milligram per day. Fortified cereals alone may not provide enough. Vitamin B_{12} helps keep the nervous system and red blood cells healthy. It's also needed to make DNA, which is why it's especially important that pregnant and nursing women have enough of it. Its deficiency can cause severe anemia and over the long term can lead to nerve malfunction with numbness and tingling in the hands and feet, poor balance, impaired memory, and depression. B_{12} deficiency can also raise blood levels of homocysteine, a marker for increased risk of heart disease or stroke. If you are committed to being a vegetarian, make sure to have your blood tested to measure your B_{12} level at least once a year.

HEART MURMUR

. . . .

When to Fix a Leaky Heart Valve

THE HEART CONTAINS FOUR VALVES whose functions include (1) directing the flow of blood from the right side of the heart into the lungs, (2) allowing blood from the left side of the heart to be pumped to the rest of the body, and (3) ensuring that blood flows normally within the heart itself. These valves are vulnerable to a variety of diseases and degenerative changes. They become narrowed, so that blood cannot easily pass through them and therefore backs up, or they don't close properly after opening, in which case blood that has been expelled from a particular heart chamber leaks back through them. In both cases, the heart must work harder to compensate for the abnormal flow—or lack of it. In time, its function is affected.

The mitral and aortic are the two valves most likely to become "stuck" or to leak. The mitral valve separates the left atrium (the upper chamber in the left side of the heart that receives freshly oxygenated blood from the lungs) from the left ventricle (the lower chamber from which this blood is pumped to the rest of the body). The normal mitral valve opens wide to allow blood to leave the left atrium and enter the left ventricle, and then it closes tightly so that none of this blood leaks back into the left atrium. However, when the valve fails to seal, every time the left ventricle contracts to pump its blood out to the rest of the body, some blood flows back into the left atrium. (This condition is called mitral regurgitation, a fancy word for "leak.") The increased volume that the left atrium now holds causes it to enlarge. The left ventricle eventually enlarges too because it has to pump harder in order to expel the now reduced amount of blood it has for the rest of the body since some of it has been "wasted" by returning to the left atrium through the leaky mitral valve.

The characteristic murmur the doctor hears with the stethoscope suggests a leaky mitral valve. The diagnosis is confirmed, and the problem's severity is evaluated by an echocardiogram.

If the mitral valve leak is substantial, you need antibiotics whenever you visit the dentist or undergo any invasive procedure or surgery in which bacteria can enter the bloodstream. Normal heart valves can deal with the presence of these organisms in the circulation. However, when a heart valve is damaged for whatever reason, its blood supply is not as abundant as when there is a normal valve, so bacteria can infect it and cause bacterial endocarditis, a potentially fatal infection. Antibiotics prevent this from happening.

It can take years for a leaky mitral valve to cause symptoms or significantly affect cardiac function. Doctors evaluate such patients at regular intervals to determine whether the left ventricle is enlarging or weakening to the point that it no longer pumps blood efficiently, and to tell whether the blood leaking into the atrium is backing up into the lungs (from where it came) and causing them to become congested. When the regurgitation is severe and the patient is short of breath even with minimal exertion, or when the heart is enlarging substantially, the valve may need to be repaired or replaced.

The decision as to when to do this is sometimes difficult. No one wants an operation unless it's really necessary. But of this you may be sure: Although mitral regurgitation may remain stable for years or worsen only slowly, it never gets better and never clears up on its own. Various medications can improve the shortness of breath or deal with an irregular heart rhythm and other complications of this condition, but they do not correct the structural alterations in the valve itself.

Traditionally, doctors do not recommend surgery until the leaky valve has begun to weaken the heart muscle. Once that has happened, the problem can be corrected by repairing or replacing the valve. Although inserting a brand-new one halts further progression of heart failure and improves symptoms, it creates several inconveniences for the patient. For example, if the new valve is a mechanical one, blood clots can form on it and then travel to the brain and cause a stroke. This can be prevented by taking blood-thinning medications (anticoagulants) that must be continued for the rest of the patient's life. One way of avoiding this is to use valves usually taken from cows or pigs. These bioprosthetic valves do not require anticoagulation, but they are not suitable for every patient and do not have the life span of the mechanical variety.

HERE'S WHAT'S NEW

Doctors at the Mayo Clinic have a special interest in techniques to repair a leaky mitral valve, because 40 years ago, one of their senior heart surgeons, Dwight McGoon, developed a technique to fix such a diseased valve rather than replace it. Researchers there recently reviewed the long-term results in 3,200 mitral valve operations done at their institution. They compared the risks and the outcomes of fixing the valve with replacing it to determine which was preferable and when best to perform the surgery. According to their statistics, 90 percent of patients with severe mitral leak eventually need to have something done about it. And the outlook is much better when the problem is corrected *before* symptoms appear. If one waits for heart failure to appear before operating, the long-term results are "dismal."

The Mayo specialists also suggest that the valve be *repaired* rather than replaced. The 10-year survival rate of patients whose valves were repaired was 70 percent, compared with only 50 percent among those who had replacements. Again, patients whose valves were repaired *before* their hearts had weakened were more likely to live longer: Their 10-year survival rate was 72 percent. Patients whose echocardiograms showed evidence of decreased function—regardless of whether symptoms were present—had only a 32 percent survival rate. The risk of death from the operation for valve repair was less than 1 percent among patients under 75 years of age.

THE BOTTOM LINE

Cardiologists and heart surgeons at the Mayo Clinic now recommend that leaking mitral valves be *repaired early—before the onset of symptoms.* This represents an important change of opinion, since previously the approach was to wait for symptoms to appear before operating. They prefer to repair the valve, rather than replace it, for several reasons: It avoids the need for blood-thinning medications, which carry with them the risk of life-threatening bleeding; mechanical valves are more likely to become infected or form clots that can break away, travel to the brain, and cause strokes; and, most important, the 10-year survival rate of patients whose valves were repaired was much greater than that of those who had valves replaced.

If you are one of the many thousands of people with severe mitral regurgitation and you are following a wait-and-see approach before having surgery, discuss these findings with your doctor. Don't wait for symptoms. Early repair may prolong and even save your life. However, and this is extremely important, choose your hospital and surgeon very carefully. Make sure your doctor has experience repairing mitral valves. Not all heart surgeons do. Finally, remember that Mayo's findings refer only to *severe* mitral regurgitation and do not apply to leaks that are minor or only moderate—a difference that's easily discernible with the echocardiogram.

HERNIA

. . . .

Surgical Options

HERNIAS OCCUR MOSTLY in children and men, but they can occur in women as well. Correcting a congenital hernia is one of the most frequently done operations on newborns. An inguinal hernia (in the groin area) is one of the most common potential reasons that people of any age need surgery.

Inguinal hernias occur in adults when the membrane (called the peritoneum) that lines the abdominal cavity and separates it from the groin stretches and ruptures, allowing the intestines and other organs to drop into the groin cavity. This is usually due to repeated straining, or lifting heavy objects, and sometimes during pregnancy. A hernia does not always cause a bulge and may only be detected in men during a physical exam when the doctor puts his finger in the scrotal sac and the patient coughs. The doctor then feels a protrusion against the examining finger. Whether or not he or she recommends surgery depends on how easily the protrusion can be pushed back and whether the hernia is causing symptoms. If the doctor concludes that a loop of bowel could become trapped within the hernia, surgery is imperative.

In the old days, most hernias were repaired by sewing together the edges of the healthy muscle tissues in order to close the gap in the damaged membrane, an operation called herniorrhaphy. But more recently, doctors have been performing a hernioplasty using a mesh patch of synthetic material (Dacron, Teflon) that is sewn over the weakened area after the hernia has been pushed back into place. The patch decreases the tension on the weakened abdominal wall and reduces the chances of the hernia recurring. This procedure requires a 3- or 4-inch incision, is done under local anesthesia, and the patient usually goes home later the same day.

Hernias are now also repaired through the "keyhole" procedure called laparoscopy. Two little holes (ports) are made in the operative area through which the surgeon inserts the instruments, as well as a small (1-centimeter-long) incision into which a tiny camera is inserted so that the surgeon can see where to place the mesh. This approach results in a slightly faster recovery than the open procedure; there is less restriction on activity afterward, and most patients are back to work and free of pain in days rather than weeks.

Although there are some advantages to repairing a hernia with laparoscopy, they are not very significant. What's more, laparoscopy requires general anesthesia while the open repair can be done under local.

HERE'S WHAT'S NEW

Until now, there has been no study comparing the *long-term* outcome of laparoscopic hernia repair with open repair. Doctors at 14

Veterans Affairs medical centers throughout the country compared the results of the two techniques among 2,000 men. They found that those who had undergone the laparoscopic surgery did indeed recover a little more quickly and had somewhat less pain during the first two postoperative weeks. However, their hernias were more likely to recur, and they were also more apt to suffer serious postoperative complications than men who'd had the open surgery. In fact, there were two postoperative deaths in the laparoscopic group and none with the conventional procedures.

The reason for this discrepancy is one that is becoming more commonplace as new techniques are introduced and embraced before those who perform them have acquired enough experience (see page 56). The poorest outcomes occurred in the hands of surgeons who had done the fewest operations. Patients of highly experienced surgeons—that is, those who had done more than 250 laparoscopic inguinal repairs—did as well as those who had the open procedure. So the open technique is superior to laparoscopy only because more surgeons really know how to do it, in contrast to the laparoscopic procedure that they haven't yet mastered.

THE BOTTOM LINE

If you have an inguinal hernia that needs fixing, you should know that there are two different surgical ways to do it. The first and older one, the open operation, involves making a small incision near the groin and introducing a mesh to close the hole between the abdomen and the groin. It's quick and easy, and you can go home the same day. The other method is the laparoscopic technique, in which the incision is avoided. It's a little quicker, you have slightly less pain, and it allows you to get back to work a day or two sooner.

The problem is that these results depend on the surgeon's experience and skill. Unless the doctor has performed this operation literally hundreds of times, the outcome is not as good as that of the older, open procedure. You're apt to have more complications and more recurrences. I personally prefer the open procedure mainly because it does not require general anesthesia. But if you favor the laparoscopic method, it's very important to ask your surgeon how many operations he or she has done this way before you sign the consent form.

HERPES

* * * * * * * * *

Keep It to Yourself

GENITAL HERPES (also called HSV-2 infection) is one of the three most prevalent sexually transmitted diseases in the United States. It currently affects at least 50 million people, more women than men. Infection with genital herpes occurs at the site of sexual contact through breaks in the skin or in moist areas such as the mouth, anus, or vagina, and in the male urethra at the tip of the penis. Characteristic blisters and sores may develop at the site of entry. However, when these lesions do not develop, those infected may be unaware of it and become unwitting reservoirs of the disease. These eruptions, when they do occur, are painful for a few days and then become shallow sores that may persist for as long as 3 weeks. The initial infection may also be accompanied by flulike symptoms.

The herpes simplex virus can also cause cold sores on the lips and in the mouth, which you can transmit to your partner's genital area. After the sores (wherever they appear) clear up, they return unpredictably—sometimes several times a year or, if you're lucky, only now and then. Although herpes is rarely a threat to life, it does leave you more vulnerable to infection by HIV, the virus that causes AIDS. It also can cause serious health consequences in newborns, of which some 1,000 are infected by their mothers every year.

Although scientists are working to develop a vaccine to prevent genital herpes, there is currently no cure. After the virus enters your body, it's there for good. Even though the sores may not return for a while after the initial ones clear up, the virus hibernates in nerve cells until the next outbreak. There are, however, several antiviral drugs that relieve the symptoms of herpes, shorten the duration of the outbreaks, and, if taken in a low dose on an ongoing basis, can reduce the number of recurrences.

One of the major problems with this disease is its transmission between an infected partner and one who isn't. Obviously, if you have herpes, you should abstain from sex with someone who is not infected while you have any visible lesions. But unfortunately, you also can transmit the disease even in the absence of such lesions. And condoms are not entirely protective either.

HERE'S WHAT'S NEW

Researchers at the Fred Hutchinson Cancer Research Center and the University of Washington, both in Seattle, have found that the antiviral drug valacyclovir, marketed as Valtrex, when taken once a day on an ongoing basis can reduce the risk of spreading HSV to an uninfected sex partner by 48 percent. These pills cost about $3.50, and possible side effects include a very low incidence of headache, nausea, and kidney problems.

THE BOTTOM LINE

There is no sure way to avoid transmitting your genital herpes virus to an uninfected partner. However, you can significantly reduce the risk by doing the following:

- Avoid sex if you have any visible sores.

- Take one Valtrex tablet every day whether or not such sores are present.

- Use a condom. Although this is not always effective—it only protects the areas it covers—it does reduce the risk.

- Finally, regardless of the title of this piece, full disclosure of your disease to your partner is the right thing to do.

HIGH BLOOD PRESSURE

· · · · · · · · ·

When You Can't Lower It

THERE ARE MANY WAYS to normalize an elevated blood pressure—and it's extremely important to do so. Untreated high blood pressure accelerates the formation of plaques that obstruct arteries anywhere in the body (hardening of the arteries), which can eventually lead to a heart attack, stroke, or damage to other organs. There are many ways to lower blood pressure: lifestyle changes such as reducing salt intake, losing weight, exercising, and taking medication.

In the old days, drugs to treat high blood pressure usually caused intolerable symptoms, everything from profound fatigue to impotence. Today, however, there is an abundance of effective medications that easily and painlessly bring the blood pressure down to the desired level of less than 140/90.

Recent studies have shown that the most effective medications are the older and least expensive water pills (diuretics)—Diuril (chlorothiazide) or Hydrodiuril (hydrochlorothiazide). They not only lower the pressure effectively but also result in fewer strokes and heart attacks than are observed with other blood-pressure-lowering drugs. However, thiazide diuretics can cause a drop in the potassium level, resulting in weakness or cardiac rhythm disturbances, especially if you're also taking other heart medications. That's why you're advised to eat a potassium-rich banana, drink orange juice, or even take potassium supplements if you're on a thiazide diuretic.

Most people with high blood pressure need more than one drug to normalize it. These include the following:

- Angiotensin converting enzyme (ACE) inhibitors such as Vasotec (enalapril)

- Angiotensin receptor blockers (ARB) such as Cozaar (losartan) or Avapro (irbesartan)

- Beta-blockers such as Tenormin (atenolol), Coreg (carvedilol), or Toprol (metoprolol)

- Calcium channel blockers (of which there are three different subgroups—Norvasc (amlodipine), Cardizem (diltiazem), or Calan (verapamil)

The great majority of hypertensive patients respond to some combination of these drugs.

HERE'S WHAT'S NEW

There is another kind of diuretic in addition to the commonly used thiazides. Called spironolactone (Aldactone), it reduces water and salt retained in the body, but unlike other diuretics, it does not lower potassium and may, in fact, increase it. Also available as Inspra (eplerenone), this agent is especially useful when the hypertension is accompanied by heart failure and fluid retention. Researchers at the University of Alabama at Birmingham found that adding a small amount of spironolactone (12.5 to 50 milligrams a day) further reduced resistant high blood pressure by an average of 21 millimeters in the top figure (systolic pressure) and 14 millimeters in the lower number (diastolic pressure) within 6 weeks.

THE BOTTOM LINE

If therapeutic doses of a combination of blood-pressure-lowering drugs have not dropped your elevated readings to the desired level, speak to your doctor about adding a small dose of spironolactone. It's a safe and effective way to achieve normal levels.

HIGH
CHOLESTEROL

· · · · · · · · · ·

Lipid Lowdown

WHEN I WAS A MEDICAL STUDENT, we were taught that cholesterol is a vital component of our sex hormones. That's it! There was no mention of its involvement with arteriosclerosis, plaques, narrowed arteries, heart attacks, and strokes. (Incidentally, in those days, high blood pressure was also considered benign unless it was causing symptoms such as headache or nosebleed. This was universal dogma.) Over the years, however, we came to understand the relationship of cholesterol and vascular disease as more and more data became available linking diet and elevated cholesterol to heart attacks and stroke. The resulting change of opinion has been gradual but continuous.

Until just a few years ago, the definition of "high" cholesterol was any number above 300. That eventually dropped to 250, but it soon

171

became clear that this level also was too high. The upper limit of "normal" is now widely accepted as 200. (I predict that it will soon be even lower than that.)

Along with the revision of what constitutes normal *total* cholesterol, we have begun to fractionate our cholesterol readings so as to include the values of its two major components—low-density lipoprotein (LDL), the "bad" cholesterol; and high-density lipoprotein (HDL), the "good" cholesterol. The former makes plaques; the latter protects against their formation. Initially, the focus was on HDL, and lab reports were usually expressed in terms of the HDL/LDL ratio. The greater that number the better, because it meant (for those of you not mathematically inclined) that the HDL was nice and high while the LDL was low.

More recently, the focus has been on the LDL level for which the recommended target numbers have been dropping. The upper limit of normal used to be 130, then it was lowered to anything less than 100.

HERE'S WHAT'S NEW

According to the results of a study reported in the *New England Journal of Medicine,* an LDL reading hovering around 100 is not good enough for anyone with established heart disease or a vulnerability to it. In a groundbreaking study of men and women who had been admitted to the hospital with heart problems and whose cholesterol was being treated, those who had received doses of a statin called Lipitor (atorvastatin) high enough to lower their LDL levels to about 60, lived longer and enjoyed better cardiovascular health than those whose average number was reduced to 95 (heretofore considered optimal). Patients with the lower figure were 30 percent less likely to have chronic chest pain and had a 14 percent lower chance of needing a blocked artery opened.

THE BOTTOM LINE

You should be as familiar with your lipid profile—the cholesterol pattern in the blood—as you are with your blood pressure reading. Both are important indicators for vascular disease, notably stroke and heart attacks—and both can be normalized, if necessary. If you are currently being treated with a lipid-lowering medication, be it a statin drug or some other therapy, ask what your cholesterol, HDL, and LDL numbers are. Your therapy should be adjusted so that your total cholesterol is kept below 200 and your LDL as low as it can go (especially if you already have heart trouble or are vulnerable to it).

Should Your Child Be Tested for It?

ACCORDING TO THE AMERICAN ACADEMY OF PEDIATRICS, up to one-third of American children, from age 2 through the teenage years, have high cholesterol levels. They also consume more of the dangerous saturated fatty acids than do kids in most other countries.

HERE'S WHAT'S NEW

Given the emphasis on normalizing cholesterol by diet, drugs, or both, increasing attention is being paid to recognizing and treating elevated levels in children as well as adults. That's because we know from autopsies performed on children who died accidentally and young soldiers who were killed in the Korean and Vietnam Wars that the buildup of plaque in the arteries starts in childhood. We also know that kids with high blood cholesterol levels have more fatty streaking (the forerunner of arteriosclerosis) in their arteries.

The guidelines may vary somewhat as to the specifics among the various professional organizations, but the message remains the same. Early detection of abnormal blood fats (that means cholesterol) is important. The American Heart Association (AHA) has recently recommended that abnormally high cholesterol should be treated as early as possible and that we should begin measuring children's blood cholesterol at age 5 (and their blood pressure at age 3). The American Academy of Pediatrics goes even further. It advocates cholesterol screening for children age 2 or older if their grandparents or parents developed heart or vascular disease prematurely, or if either parent has a cholesterol reading of 240 or higher. The information about grandparents is especially important because the parents and siblings might not yet be old enough to have developed heart disease.

According to the AHA, total cholesterol levels in children ages 2 to 19 years should be less than 170, and LDL levels should not exceed 110. Although we do not yet have evidence that lowering these cholesterol levels so early in life reduces risk later on, all the available data from adults suggest that it does. Even though high cholesterol levels during childhood often become normal in adult life, the U.S. National Cholesterol Education Program recommends cholesterol-lowering drugs for children over age 10 when the LDL (the "bad" cholesterol) remains high even after they've changed their diets. The most common class of such drugs, the statins, have recently been found to be safe and are approved for use in children who need them, especially those with an inherited form of high cholesterol. One study involving 173 children between the ages of 10 and 17 found that after 48 weeks on the drug, there was no adverse effect on growth or development of puberty. Studies of longer duration are obviously needed.

THE BOTTOM LINE

Children with the risk factors described above should have their lipids screened after they are 2 years old. (Since the normal diet of children younger than 2 years is high in fat and therefore high in cholesterol, it is not appropriate to test them.)

There is no agreement exactly when to check the cholesterol levels of children who are not at high risk. I happen to believe that it's a good idea to test everyone to identify those with high cholesterol. In such cases, educating them about eating and exercise habits that lower cholesterol levels can be started early in life. The main arguments against such testing are cost, as well as the fact that high cholesterol levels do not always persist into adulthood, and that *all* children be educated anyway about healthy diet and lifestyle, regardless of cholesterol levels.

If your child is found to have high cholesterol, everyone else in your family should also be checked.

WHAT THE DOCTOR ORDERED?

THE STATIN MIRACLE ● Every now and then, a medication that was originally developed to treat or prevent a specific illness or symptoms is found to do much more than was expected. Aspirin is a good example of such a drug. Introduced a little more than a century ago to relieve mild pain and to lower fever, over the years it has gone on to greater things. Because it reduces the tendency of the blood to clot, it offers powerful protection against heart disease and stroke. It also lowers the risk of certain cancers. Who knows what other effects it will turn out to have?

The statin family of drugs, introduced for the specific purpose of normalizing an abnormal cholesterol profile, has reduced the incidence of heart attacks and strokes, regardless of the cholesterol level of those who take it.

There are many statins on the market—the best-known brands are Lipitor (atorvastatin), Zocor (simvastatin), Lescol (fluvastatin), Pravachol (pravastatin), Mevacor (lovastatin), and Crestor (rosuvastatin). They all lower total cholesterol levels and/or increase the good HDL and lower the bad LDL, although the extent to which they do so varies.

HERE'S WHAT'S NEW • The statin drugs have been found to have benefits far beyond normalizing cholesterol levels. These other effects (described below) seem to stem from their anti-inflammatory properties. Many doctors now believe that inflammation, often silent, in a particular area or organ in the body is the first step in the development of many our most deadly diseases—Alzheimer's, cancer, or the sudden obstruction of a critical artery in the heart or the brain. The statins appear to reduce that inflammation.

Here are some of the diseases that can be helped by cholesterol-lowering drugs. Some of these effects have been confirmed; others are still being investigated.

Heart rhythm disturbances. The statins lower the incidence of abnormal cardiac rhythm. Canadian researchers found that statins given to patients with documented heart disease resulted in a 39 percent decrease in death from cardiac causes and 36 percent fewer noncardiac deaths. This benefit is believed due to the anti-arrhythmic effect of these drugs.

Another study showed that patients with the very common arrhythmia called atrial fibrillation also benefited from statin therapy. After a 2-year follow-up of men and women with atrial fibrillation that came and went (and high cholesterol levels), 60 percent of those treated with a statin drug remained in normal heart rhythm as compared with only 16 percent of those not receiving these drugs. It's not clear whether these beneficial effects are due to a specific action on the rhythm centers of the heart or the control of plaque formation within the arteries of the heart associated with elevated cholesterol. Whatever the mechanism, the end results are very impressive.

Nonischemic cardiomyopathy. This is a form of heart disease in which the heart is enlarged, thickened, or stiff. The result is heart failure—a reduced ability to pump blood. Nonischemic cardiomyopathy is often accompanied by a serious heart-rhythm disturbance. According to the American Heart Association's Heart Disease and Stroke Statistics, cardiomyopathy was the cause of more than 27,000 deaths in 2003, especially among African Americans. Japanese doctors studied 63 patients with heart failure caused by this disorder for 14 weeks, during which time they found that giving them a statin drug strengthened the heart muscle and improved its function.

Peripheral vascular disease with intermittent claudication. In this condition, plaque formations obstruct the arteries of the leg so that walking causes pain in the calf muscles. Researchers at the University of Pennsylvania in Philadelphia treated 354 patients with this disorder—some with statins, others with placebos. After a year, they found that 63 percent of the statin-treated group was able to walk greater distances without pain while only 38 percent of those on placebos reported any improvement. The benefit from the statins is attributed to the reduction in the size of the obstructing arterial plaques.

Mental health. In two large studies, statins were found to improve psychological well-being. Researchers at Harvard found that patients who had been taking one of these medications (with the exception of Pravachol) for 4 years were less depressed and anxious than subjects not taking them. These results are likely due to a chemical antidepressant effect on the brain by these agents.

In another study of men and women with heart disease, the risk of depression was 60 percent lower in those receiving a statin. The investigators explain the antidepressant effect in the cardiac patients in this study by the fact that the statins improved the course of heart disease, which contributed to a better overall quality of life.

Multiple sclerosis (MS). The most common neurological disorder among young adults, this disease results from the destruction of the myelin sheath that surrounds nerve fibers. Scar tissue then forms in the areas of the central nervous system where the myelin is damaged. Without myelin, nerves lose their capacity to transmit electrical impulses. This causes a wide variety of symptoms leading progressively to debilitation—many patients eventually end up in a wheelchair.

Although there are many medications that control the symptoms of MS and the frequency of the relapses that characterize it, there is no cure. Several studies suggest, however, that the statin drugs may improve symptoms presumably by virtue of their anti-inflammatory effects. Research in the United States and abroad has reported as much as a 44 percent decrease in the number of brain lesions in patients with this disease.

Cancer. Researchers in the Netherlands found that the overall risk of developing cancer was reduced by about 20 percent in people who took a statin for 4 years or more. This risk returned to baseline within 6 months after the drugs were stopped. More recently a study at the University of Michigan in Ann Arbor compared 1,849 people who had colon cancer with 1,959 who did not. Those taking a statin for at least 5 years were 50 percent less likely to have developed this malignancy. The researchers believe this benefit is related to the anti-inflammatory properties of these drugs rather than their cholesterol-lowering properties.

Osteoporosis. Statin use resulted in a 57 percent reduction in the rate of hip factures and 31 percent fewer nonspine fractures in trials done in the Netherlands and at the University of California, San Francisco. Scientists believe that the statins work much like the bisphosphonates—Actonel (risedronate) and Fosamax (alendronate)—conventionally used to treat osteoporosis and prevent the reabsorption of bone.

Death after major surgery. A study from Baystate Medical Center in Springfield, Massachusetts, analyzed the postoperative course of more than 780,000 patients who underwent major noncardiac surgery in the years 2000 and 2001. The death rate for men and women who had been treated with a statin for at least 2 years prior to surgery was 2.13 percent as opposed to 3.05 percent for nonusers. This lower postoperative death rate in people who take a statin drug is thought to result from the action of the statins on arterial plaques in the heart.

Alzheimer's disease. An increasing number of studies have shown that the statins are effective in the management of this disease. In a study of almost 57,000 patients at three hospitals, doctors at the Boston University School of Medicine reported in the *Lancet* that taking statins reduced the risk of Alzheimer's by 70 percent. This benefit has also been observed in animal experiments.

Diabetes. People with diabetes can benefit dramatically by incorporating the statin drugs into their treatment regimen. A study last year showed that using Zocor cut the risk of heart attack and stroke by one-third among men and women with diabetes.

More recently, a study sponsored by Diabetes U.K., Britain's Department of Health, and Pfizer U.K. (the maker of Lipitor) revealed that a 10-milligram dose of Lipitor reduced cardiovascular events by 37 percent in people with diabetes who had no previous history of cardiovascular disease, while the incidence of stroke fell by 48 percent. The investigators involved in this trial conclude that doctors should now consider giving the statin drugs routinely to all patients with diabetes, regardless of their cholesterol level.

Eye health. Researchers at the University of Alabama at Birmingham found that men taking a statin drug had a 50 percent lower incidence of macular degeneration (see page 108), a very common age-related cause of vision loss. (Aspirin protects against it, too.) The mechanism by which the statins afford such protection is not clear, but it is presumed to be their anti-inflammatory effect.

These same researchers believe that the use of statins also reduces the risk for open-angle glaucoma, an eye disease associated with increased ocular pressure that affects roughly 3 million Americans, half of whom don't know they have it. When examining the records of 667 men age 50 or older, they found that those who had used statins for 24 months or more had a significantly lower incidence of glaucoma (as did the men who took other cholesterol-lowering drugs).

Rheumatoid arthritis. Patients with rheumatoid arthritis who are given specific drugs to treat their disease usually respond in 6 to 8 joints among the 12 to 15 that are swollen when the therapy is started. Researchers at the Glasgow Royal Infirmary in Scotland gave 116 patients with rheumatoid arthritis a daily 40-milligram dose of Lipitor for 6 months and found a reduction of swelling in an average of 3 joints. This is a definite response, albeit a modest one. It is nevertheless important because patients with rheumatoid arthritis are at greater risk for heart attack and stroke. Giving them a statin (in this case, Lipitor) not only provides some pain relief but also reduces their vulnerability to a vascular event—a noteworthy combination of effects.

Overall, the statins are safe and effective. But remember that there is a little poison in every medication. No active agent, whether herbal or prescription, is entirely free of side effects. A small number of statin users develop liver function abnormalities. However, these clear up when the drug is stopped. That's why you should have your blood checked 2 months after starting a statin, and every 6 months to a year thereafter. These medications can also cause muscle pain that may force you to stop taking them. One more serious consequence recently reported but happily quite rare is a lupuslike syndrome. Apparently, statins (in this case, Pravachol) can result in the production of antibodies that produce a rash similar to that seen in cases of lupus, an autoimmune disorder. This too clears up several months after the drug is stopped.

The statin drugs are so effective, generally so well tolerated, and have so many obvious (and potential) benefits that there is pressure on the FDA to make them available in lower doses over the counter. The FDA has not decided whether to do so. Zocor can already be purchased without a prescription in the United Kingdom.

THE BOTTOM LINE • The lipid-lowering statin drugs reduce the incidence of heart attack and stroke, regardless of whether or not cholesterol levels are abnormal. This suggests that these drugs act in other ways in addition to controlling a wide variety of disorders, including cardiac arrhythmias, diseases of the heart muscle (cardiomyopathy), clogged arteries in the legs, depression and anxiety, multiple sclerosis, cancer, osteoporosis, Alzheimer's disease, diabetes, glaucoma, and macular degeneration. Although some of the evidence is preliminary, it is very compelling. If you suffer from any of these disorders, discuss with your doctor whether you should take a statin drug along with the specific therapy for your disease.

HIV/AIDS

....

One Way to Cut the Risk

WHETHER OR NOT TO CIRCUMCISE male infants has been hotly debated over the ages. There is an organization currently lobbying Congress to have the practice outlawed in the United States. The arguments pro and con are largely cultural or religious, rather than medical. One wag remarked to me that those in favor of circumcision were obviously optimists, prepared to cut the male member short before they knew how long it would be!

I am neutral on the subject of circumcision. I was never asked for my permission before it was done to me at the age of 7 days. I can't remember the details, but it could not have been pleasant.

From a purely medical and health standpoint, here are some of the facts on which doctors generally agree about circumcision. It results in:

- Fewer urinary tract infections

- Reduced risk of cancer of the penis

- Decreased likelihood of cervical cancer in a man's sexual partners

- Fewer inflammatory conditions involving the foreskin

Given these observations, one would expect that, religious opinions aside, the medical profession would favor the procedure. Not so. Virtually every professional medical organization from America to Australia has concluded that there is no absolute medical indication for routine circumcision of the newborn. Talk about a non sequitur!

HERE'S WHAT'S NEW

Researchers at Johns Hopkins Hospital in Baltimore have found that circumcision protects against HIV infection. It had previously been speculated that the foreskin, not the penis itself, harbors the organisms responsible for a variety of sexually transmitted diseases, notably the human papillomavirus (HPV), which causes cervical cancer. This was presumed to be the reason why female sexual partners of circumcised men have a reduced incidence of this cancer.

These observations were made between 1993 and 2000 in some 2,300 men attending a sexually transmitted disease clinic in India. All the subjects were HIV-negative when the study began. Some had been circumcised; others had not. At its conclusion, there were six to eight times fewer HIV infections among the circumcised men than the others. (There were no cultural or religious differences between the two groups.) Circumcision did not affect other sexually transmitted diseases such as herpes, syphilis, and gonorrhea.

The doctors speculate that circumcision protects against HIV because the foreskin contains cells with HIV receptors that are the primary entry site for the virus into the penis. This is the ninth consecutive study to demonstrate the protective effect of removing the foreskin.

THE BOTTOM LINE

I don't expect that these findings will necessarily convince most young parents-to-be to have their sons circumcised. No one expects his or her child to contract AIDS. However, from an epidemiologic and public health viewpoint, until we find a vaccine or cure for HIV, circumcising newborn boys may be one way to help reduce the incidence of this scourge.

New Tests, Faster Results

ONE IN EVERY FOUR of the 900,000 people infected with HIV in this country is not aware of it. Despite "being careful" and practicing "safer sex," statistics show that any of the following characteristics can expose you to the risk of AIDS. You should be tested for HIV if:

- You have been sexually active with three or more sexual partners in the last 12 months.
- You received a blood transfusion between 1977 and 1985 (when donor blood could not be screened for the AIDS virus) or a sexual partner received a transfusion and later tested positive for HIV.
- You are not sure about your sexual partner's risk behavior.

- You are a male and have had sex with other males at any time since 1977.

- Any of your male sexual partners has had sex with another male since 1977.

- You have used street drugs by injection since 1977, sharing needles or other equipment.

- You are female and have a sexually transmitted disease, including pelvic inflammatory disease.

- You are a health-care worker with potential exposure to blood on the job.

- You are a woman and want to make sure you are not infected with HIV before becoming pregnant.

Even if none of the above apply to you, get yourself tested for HIV if you are at all worried that you may have it. If you remain unaware of your infection, and so neither seek nor receive any treatment for it, you're not only harming yourself but also endangering anyone you unwittingly expose to this disease.

Being tested for HIV has always meant waiting for as long as 2 weeks for the results, whether it was from your own doctor or from a clinic. That's a long time to stew, especially if you're anxious about the results. And it may be the reason that a substantial number of men and women who test positive for AIDS at public clinics do not come back for their results.

In the 2004 edition of *Breakthrough Health,* I reported on two new rapid HIV tests that had recently become available. Both are accurate and provide results in just a few minutes. Getting a quick answer to an HIV test is extremely important. For example, a pregnant woman at high risk for passing the virus to her unborn child can now have her HIV status determined rapidly, and drugs can be administered right then and there to prevent her from infecting her child during delivery.

HERE'S WHAT'S NEW

Two more tests that provide the answer virtually immediately are on the market. The first, made in Ireland and called the Uni-Gold Recombigen HIV test, gives you the result in 10 minutes. It is available overseas for you to do in the privacy of your own home (and actively advertised there for that purpose). But in the United States, the FDA has restricted the use of Uni-Gold to laboratory professionals in clinics and other facilities with an adequate quality-assurance program—the worry being that if improperly done and interpreted, a quick but wrong answer might do more harm than good. This test is virtually 100 percent accurate, and one of its conveniences is that it requires just a drop of blood, not a vial obtained from your vein. Each test kit costs the doctor or clinic about $10. Just to be sure, all positive tests require follow-up confirmation with the conventional blood test. But if you're negative, you can go out and celebrate!

The second test, OraQuick, is also virtually 100 percent accurate, provides the results while you're waiting, and doesn't even require blood. It is so easy to do that the government allows it to be used in doctor's offices as well as in community and HIV counseling centers. A technician wipes your gums with a treated cotton swab that picks up cells lining the mouth. The swab is then inserted into a vial. Twenty minutes later, if you are infected, a reddish purple line appears in a window on the vial. Again, if you test positive, you will have your blood tested just to be sure.

You should be very careful where you buy these HIV antibody

tests. According to the Federal Trade Commission (FTC), one such test, the Discreet HIV antibody test kit, sold since 2001 by two Canadian-based Web sites, www.AIDSHIVTest.com and Discreettest.com, is wildly inaccurate. The FTC recommends that anyone who has used this kit (at least 3,000 were shipped to the United States by Federal Express in 2003) should be retested immediately.

Currently, the only home HIV test approved for home use in this country is called the Home Access Express HIV-1 Test System. You can buy it at some pharmacies for about $50. I don't see much point in doing so, because you don't test the sample yourself; instead you must send it to a lab for analysis.

THE BOTTOM LINE
There's no need anymore to wait days and weeks for the outcome of an HIV test. There are several new ways to have it done at a clinic or your doctor's office by just pricking your finger or having your gums swabbed. They can tell you accurately, easily, very quickly, and at little cost whether you are infected with HIV. But whenever one of these rapid-fire tests comes back positive, you will be required to have the old-fashioned blood test to confirm it. That's reasonable, given the implications of a positive test. However, these new techniques provide you with a quick answer that ends an agonizing wait.

The Best Treatment Cocktail

THERE ARE SOME FACTS about AIDS that have not changed since the 2004 volume of *Breakthrough Health*. The disease continues to spread worldwide, and the greatest problem remains in sub-Saharan

Africa. Almost 1 million Americans are afflicted by this disease, mostly men between ages 25 and 44.

AIDS is caused by HIV, which impairs the function of the immune system, leaving the body defenseless against infections that it can normally overcome. As a result, patients usually die from what are called opportunistic diseases: *Pneumocystis carinii* pneumonia (PCP), which affects the lungs; Kaposi's sarcoma, which involves the skin; and a variety of other viral, fungal, and bacterial infections that spread through the intestinal tract, brain, and nervous system.

There is no cure for AIDS, but you can and must avoid it. It is spread among adults mainly by sexual contact, shared needles used for intravenous drugs, and now, very rarely, by blood transfusions.

If you are vulnerable to AIDS by virtue of any of these risk factors, and especially if you share needles or are a sexually active male who has sex with other men, do not ignore any of the following symptoms: an unexplained cough, fever, rash, persistent headache, unusual irritability, neurological signs and symptoms such as double vision, numbness or weakness of an arm or leg, or a stiff neck. Remember, however, that you can be harboring the AIDS virus and not have any symptoms whatsoever. I have several patients who have tested positive for HIV for as long as 12 years, yet still feel perfectly well without any other evidence of the infection.

Although there is no cure for AIDS, there are medications that can slow the progress of the disease for years, control its symptoms, and improve quality of life. These drugs, called antiretrovirals, work by making it difficult for the virus to reproduce. There are currently about 20 such HIV drugs on the market, and they lend themselves literally to hundreds of possible combinations. However, they fall into three main groups.

- Nucleoside reverse transcriptase inhibitors, such as Epivir (lamivudine) and AZT (zidovudine)

- Protease inhibitors, such as Norvir (ritonavir) and Crixivan (indinavir)

- Nonnucleoside reverse transcriptase inhibitors, such as Rescriptor (delavirdine) and Viramune (nevirapine)

These drugs yield the best results when used together.

HERE'S WHAT'S NEW

Researchers led by doctors at Harvard and Stanford universities tested several drug combinations of six different HIV medicines. Their study involved 1,000 patients at 58 hospitals and clinics in the United States and 23 in Italy. It was begun in 1998 and continued for 28 months. In treating patients newly diagnosed with AIDS, one particular three-drug "cocktail" was found to be clearly superior to other combinations. It worked better for longer, was easier to take, and suppressed the virus more quickly. The researchers also found that combining four drugs is not necessarily better than three.

On the basis of these findings, the U.S. Department of Health and Human Services has changed its guidelines for the initial treatment of HIV and recommends the three-drug combination of efavirenz (Sustiva), zidovudine (AZT), and lamivudine (Epivir). (The last two drugs can be combined in one tablet sold as Combivir.) One advantage of this particular mixture is that it enables doctors to defer treatment with the powerful class of drugs called protease inhibitors for later use if necessary. It's always good to have such an agent in reserve.

THE BOTTOM LINE

AIDS is a deadly disease for which there is currently no cure. Research, however, continues at a furious pace. If you are infected with

HIV, the more time you can buy, the greater the chance that you will one day be cured. So this is no time to be negative or fatalistic about your future. Find a doctor with special expertise in treating AIDS and then together make the decision concerning when to start therapy. But also draw your doctor's attention to this study and the combination of drugs now recommended.

HOUSEHOLD
ACCIDENTS

New Poisoning-Treatment Guidelines

In 1989, the American Academy of Pediatrics (AAP) officially recommended that every medicine cabinet should contain a 1-ounce bottle of ipecac to induce vomiting in anyone, especially a child, who had accidentally swallowed poison. Many years ago, as an emergency-room resident, I went by the book and gave ipecac to all poisoning cases. I hated to do so because the uncontrollable vomiting this drug caused often left many patients who were already scared and sick from the poison feeling even worse.

HERE'S WHAT'S NEW

The AAP has changed its position on ipecac and now advises *against* its use. Moreover, an FDA advisory committee has gone so far as to recommend not only that ipecac not be sold over the counter but that we should throw out any that remains in our drug cabinets. The reason for this dramatic reversal of opinion is that there is absolutely no evidence that ipecac does any good in poisoning cases, whether used at home or in the ER. What's more, when taken improperly, such as by someone with an eating disorder who wants to vomit to lose weight, ipecac has been known to cause complications ranging from inhaling the regurgitated material, thereby blocking the airway, to placing severe stress on an already weakened heart.

Now that ipecac is no longer in the picture, here is the latest advice on how to deal with poisoning.

- The first and obvious step is to keep all toxic substances out of the sight and reach of children.

- Always leave a poison in its original container so that it remains clear what the contents are.

- Once *any* medication has expired, throw it out.

- Never entice children to take medication by referring to it as candy.

- In the event of poisoning, call the National Capital Poison Center at (800) 222-1222. You will be connected immediately to a local facility.

- Poisons that superficially involve the skin or eyes should be diluted by running tap water over the area for 15 to 20 minutes.

- Call 911 immediately if the poisoned victim has collapsed or stopped breathing.

Activated charcoal is now the single safest and most effective antipoisoning drug. Unlike ipecac, which induces vomiting, charcoal binds to the chemicals in the stomach or intestines, preventing them from reaching the bloodstream. It is eventually excreted in the stool. For maximum effectiveness, it should be taken as soon as possible.

There is a difference of opinion, however, about whether charcoal should be taken at home or administered by a doctor in the ER through a stomach tube. We keep activated charcoal in our medicine cabinet just in case an adult should need it. Some doctors feel that because kids may have trouble swallowing it, you should simply rush them to the ER. Others, including me, recommend that you have them try to take it because the sooner it gets into the stomach and deactivates the poison, the better. But take them to the ER anyway, just in case.

THE BOTTOM LINE

Ipecac should no longer be used to treat acute poisoning in children or adults. Activated charcoal is now recommended instead. Keep some in your medicine cabinet, but go to the nearest emergency room if there is any question about a victim's response to it. In every case of poisoning, call the National Capital Poison Center at (800) 222-1222 for emergency information. If the patient is unconscious or not breathing normally, call 911 or rush him or her to the nearest ER. Most important, prevent poisoning by making sure all toxic substances are out of a child's reach.

Softer Floor, Fewer Fractures

EVERY NOW AND THEN doctors substantiate common sense and important advice with scientific research. One such study, published in the journal *Age and Ageing*, was motivated by the fact that almost 2 million hip fractures every year result in the death or disability of many elderly men and women the world over. We try to prevent these fractures by treating osteoporosis so that bones won't break as easily and by encouraging elderly people with an unstable gait to wear rubber-soled shoes and use canes and other supports when they move about.

HERE'S WHAT'S NEW

Researchers visited 34 residential nursing homes in the United Kingdom over a 2-year period and correlated the total number of falls that took place in each of them with the type of floors they had. There were a total of 6,641 falls that resulted in 222 hip fractures. The risk of a hip fracture was 78 percent lower when someone fell on a carpeted wooden floor than when they did so on a bare wooden or concrete floor, or a carpeted concrete floor. The researchers explain this difference by the fact that the carpeted wooden floors absorb much more of the shock of the fall than do the others, and so protect bones from breaking.

THE BOTTOM LINE

Although the doctors who conducted the study conclude that residents of nursing homes are typically frail and many have a tendency to fall, their observations are relevant to all seniors, no matter where they live. We can't carpet our pavements, but we can cover our floors—at home and in residential facilities for the elderly. Such a simple measure could significantly reduce the number of hip fractures and improve the quality of life for many thousands of men and women.

INTERMITTENT CLAUDICATION

. . . .

Freeze Your Arteries Open

WHEN THE ARTERIES IN YOUR LEGS become clogged (usually because of atherosclerotic plaques, which also often develop in the heart, brain, eyes, and kidneys), blood flow is reduced, and the leg muscles are deprived of oxygen. As a consequence, walking causes calf pain. These symptoms clear up soon after you rest for a few minutes, after which you are usually able to resume walking.

This scenario, called intermittent claudication, can be dealt with in a number of ways. You should continue to walk as much and as often as you can. This stimulates the formation of new blood vessels in the leg—a process called collateral circulation. In time, these new blood vessels deliver additional blood to the oxygen-deprived muscles. Walking, of course, is beneficial for many other reasons. It helps

195

you lose weight, it's good for the heart, and if you have diabetes (a common cause of vascular disease), it helps keep your blood sugar under control.

In addition to telling you to remain as active as possible, most doctors will prescribe medication to increase blood flow in the narrowed leg arteries, permitting you to walk farther before the pain sets in. I have found Pletal (cilostazol) to be the most effective such agent currently available. (However, do not use it if you also have coronary artery disease.)

If your symptoms worsen despite these conservative measures, you may be advised to have an angiogram to determine which arteries are narrowed and how severely. Depending on what the angiogram shows, there are essentially two major treatment options. In the first, the blockages can be surgically bypassed, just as they are in the heart when the coronary arteries are diseased. Veins taken from the groin area are sewn into the legs around the blocked arteries, bypassing the obstructed areas. Or you may be a candidate for angioplasty, in which a catheter with a little balloon at its end is threaded into the clogged vessel. The balloon is then inflated to compress the blockage and re-open the artery. A flexible metal sleeve, called a stent, is then inserted into the artery to keep it open.

Angioplasty of leg arteries is not usually as successful as it is in the coronary arteries. That's usually because the leg vessels are apt to be more extensively diseased and are much longer than those in the heart. As a result, in 40 to 50 percent of cases, the ballooned artery closes up (restenosis) within months after it has been opened.

HERE'S WHAT'S NEW

Researchers have developed a technique called CryoPlasty to clear blocked arteries in the extremities. It is less traumatic to the blood vessels than angioplasty, and they remain open more often and for longer.

Angioplasty and CryoPlasty are very similar. In both, a catheter is threaded into the blocked artery, and a balloon is inflated to compress the obstructing plaque and reopen the vessel. But here's the difference. In conventional angioplasty, the balloon is inflated with a salt solution, while in CryoPlasty, it is inflated with nitrous oxide—better known as laughing gas. The nitrous oxide cools the artery to a temperature of $-10°C$, freezing the plaque and causing apoptosis, a type of cell death that prevents scar formation. CryoPlasty is easier on the artery wall than angioplasty and causes less of the inflammation and scarring that blocks the vessel again. This new technique is as safe as conventional angioplasty and usually does not require the insertion of a stent.

The FDA has approved CryoPlasty, and it is now being performed in several hospitals in the United States, where the average failure or recurrence rate is about 20 percent, as compared with 40 to 50 percent with conventional angioplasty.

THE BOTTOM LINE

If blocked arteries in your legs are causing you pain when you walk, keep active and take the medication that can alleviate the symptoms. If these measures fail and the quality of your life is affected, ask your doctor about CryoPlasty. It appears to be more effective than angioplasty and is less invasive than surgery.

KIDNEY STONES

• • • • • • • • • •

Coffee and Wine Prevent Kidney Stones

EACH YEAR, KIDNEY STONES STRIKE at least 1 million Americans, mostly between the ages of 20 and 40. If you've ever had a stone, you know that the pain can be unbearable. Kidney stones form when certain constituents in the urine solidify. If you have kidney stones, the more fluids you drink, the smaller your risk of a new one forming. But does it matter *what* you drink?

HERE'S WHAT'S NEW

You can't go wrong with water, but newer research shows that apple juice and grapefruit juice *increase* the risk of kidney stones. While on the other hand, drinking an 8-ounce glass of red or white wine reduced risk by 59 percent. In another study of 81,000 women, an 8-ounce serving of regular coffee per day *lowered* the incidence by

10 percent, and the same amount of decaffeinated coffee did so by 9 percent. But as you reach for the java, remember to limit it to 2 cups a day if you are prone to kidney stones. When scientists at Washington State University in Spokane gave a group of people who had a history of kidney stones the amount of caffeine equivalent to 2 cups of coffee, they found high levels of calcium in their urine. Increased urinary calcium raises the risk of kidney stone formation.

THE BOTTOM LINE

If you have kidney stones, drink lots of fluids (except apple and grapefruit juices) and remember that drinking a glass of wine or no more than 2 cups of coffee each day reduces your chances of forming more stones.

MALE MENOPAUSE

· · · · · · · · · ·

Testosterone Replacement—What's a Guy to Do?

IN THEIR FORTIES, women begin to make less of the female hormone estrogen, and those levels continue to fall as they approach 50. During this time, menstrual periods become irregular. Once a woman goes a full year without a menstruating, she is officially considered menopausal.

There is no unanimity about whether there is also a male menopause. Those who think there is point to the fact that as men age, the level of free testosterone in their blood decreases markedly. (Free testosterone is that portion of the male hormone not bound to protein, which normally accounts for 2 percent of the total testosterone level.) According to these doctors, these low levels of free testosterone account for the diminished potency, decreased libido, depression, weight gain, fatigue, and loss of muscle and bone mass that characterize a "change of life" in men. Replacing the waning testosterone can, they believe, reverse most of these symptoms.

Other physicians disagree. They attribute most of these symptoms not to hormone levels but to midlife crisis—the consequences of all the physical and psychological factors that come together at that time in a man's life. These include fear of aging, marital problems, and empty-nest syndrome. At this time in their lives, men may also become more aware of their own mortality as their parents and many friends die. Some also have failed to achieve lifelong goals and are confronted with the realization that they may never attain them.

In addition, these middle years mark the onset of other medical problems such as heart disease, high blood pressure, diabetes, tumors, hearing and vision loss—and the side effects of the drugs to treat them—all of which contribute to depression and an impaired self-image. These experts believe that what men need to restore their well-being is not testosterone supplements but a program of regular exercise, counseling, abstinence from smoking, a reduction of alcohol intake, and when necessary, Viagra!

HERE'S WHAT'S NEW

A compromise seems to have been reached between these two polarized opinions. Although not specifically using the term *male menopause,* many doctors agree that men with very low levels of free testosterone do feel better when they take testosterone supplements.

Total testosterone levels have such a wide range (anywhere from 500 to 1,000 nanograms per deciliter) that they are of little use in making a treatment decision. The free testosterone is what counts. These levels fall not only with age but also sometimes in association with diabetes, coronary artery disease, long-term steroid therapy, and genetic factors. Investigators at the National Institute on Aging found that the less free testosterone a man has, the higher his risk of developing Alzheimer's disease. More and more doctors now agree that screening to determine the free testosterone level should be part of a middle-aged man's regular checkup.

The danger in taking testosterone simply to "feel better" if your levels are not very low is that high (as opposed to "normal") levels are associated with an increased risk of prostate cancer. Researchers at Johns Hopkins Hospital in Baltimore and the National Institute on Aging have shown that extra testosterone can promote cancer growth in the prostate. (Note, however, that total testosterone levels do not predispose to prostate cancer if the free testosterone level is normal.) Too much testosterone also thickens the blood, increases the risk of stroke, and worsens sleep apnea in men who already have it. Free testosterone should not exceed 1 to 2 percent of your total testosterone reading (and that should be between 500 and 1,000 nanograms per deciliter).

Testosterone can be replaced by pills, a topical gel, a patch, or an injection. I suggest that you avoid the pill because it has the highest incidence of side effects, the most serious of which is liver damage.

THE BOTTOM LINE

So what is a guy to do? If you are over 40 and have begun to feel "lousy," there's no harm in having your testosterone levels checked. (As my mother would have said, "Harm it can't do.") Take supplements only if the free testosterone is extremely low and if *you have specific symptoms that cannot be explained in any other way*. Remember, however, that the level to pay most attention to is free testosterone, too little of which has been implicated in vulnerability to Alzheimer's disease; too much of which indicates a greater risk for prostate cancer.

There is no treatment for high testosterone except to avoid any supplements.

OVERACTIVE BLADDER

· · · · · · · · ·

Botox—The New Miracle Drug?

MORE THAN 20 MILLION American men and women of all ages suffer from an overactive bladder. Many are too embarrassed to tell anyone about it, even their doctors. Some of these people have to empty their bladders as often as 30 and 40 times a day, and when they must do so, there's no time to look for a toilet. It's now—or flooding! As a result, many either stay home or wear diapers. The sudden intense need to urinate is sometimes followed by incontinence (uncontrollable leakage of urine) caused by involuntary bladder contractions that occur as the shrunken bladder fills with urine. For men and women with these problems, intercourse is usually painful.

Symptoms of an overactive bladder become worse as you grow older, and they are more common in women. This disorder can be caused by a variety of conditions: stroke, chronic urinary tract infection, bladder tumor, or interstitial cystitis. Here, the bladder wall is irritated, scarred, or stiff, allowing it to hold much less urine. But the kidneys couldn't care less about the bladder's problems and continue to make urine. Since the urine has to be excreted and there is no effective storage facility, it continually passes right out of the body. Patients with severe interstitial cystitis urinate as often as 60 times a day. More than 700,000 Americans, 90 percent of them women, are believed to have interstitial cystitis.

There are many ways to treat an overactive bladder—lifestyle changes, bladder retraining, and pelvic-muscle exercises, all usually combined with drug therapy. The main medications are antidepressants, which help you cope with the misery, and anticholinergic drugs, which neutralize acetylcholine, a neurotransmitter that causes the muscles to contract. Without the acetylcholine to stimulate them, the bladder muscles are less likely to cause problems. Detrol (tolterodine), whose 24-hour formulation is especially effective, is perhaps the most widely used anticholinergic. A new member of this family of drugs, called Oxytrol (oxybutynin), is said to be easier to tolerate and comes in the form of skin patch. However, all these medicines have side effects such as dry mouth and constipation that some patients find distressing over the long term. In men who also have urinary obstruction due to an enlarged prostate, anticholinergic drugs can cause acute retention of urine—and require emergency catheterization to relieve it.

HERE'S WHAT'S NEW

The anticholinergic agents mentioned above can reduce symptoms of an overactive bladder, but there is a surprising new treatment now available: tiny amounts of the toxin produced by the deadly bacterium *Clostridium botulinum,* which lives in soil. It's not nearly as famous as some other bugs like staph, strep, and *Escherichia coli* (*E. coli*), but clostridium causes several different types of diseases known collectively as botulism. The most common and important one results from the bacterial contamination of food by clostridium spores that produce a dangerous nerve toxin that causes a serious, often fatal paralytic illness.

This "poison" has become a wonder drug, marketed as Botox. Best known these days as a cosmetic product to remove facial wrinkles, it has been used for years to treat an ever-growing list of conditions (see page 206).

When used in patients with an overactive bladder, Botox paralyzes the nerves that release acetylcholine, so that the muscle is not stimulated and is less spastic. A cystoscope with a small telescope at its end is inserted through the urethra into the bladder. There are no incisions in the skin. A small needle is inserted into the bladder through which multiple injections of Botox are administered. Patients go home the same day and typically experience obvious improvement within 5 to 7 days, which usually lasts for 3 to 6 months, sometimes for as long as 9 months. When its effect wears off, you can have another treatment. Botox can also be given to patients whose bladder problems are due to neurological causes such as spinal cord injury, stroke, or multiple sclerosis, and whenever the bladder cannot contract normally and needs to be catheterized.

One of the pioneers in this application of Botox is a Houston urologist named Christopher Smith, M.D., who works at the Baylor College of Medicine.

THE BOTTOM LINE

The drugs currently available to control the troublesome symptoms of an overactive bladder do help but apparently not as well as Botox does. If you are devastated by the symptoms of an overactive bladder, ask your urologist about his or her experience with Botox. If there's any question, I suggest you call Baylor in Houston. Botox might make a big difference in your life.

What the Doctor Ordered?

OTHER BOTOX BENEFITS The horrible clostridium bug is continuing to enjoy increasing fame and popularity because when its nightmare toxin is greatly diluted and injected into various muscles and organs, it can paralyze selected nerves so that the muscles they stimulate become limp and flaccid, relieving painful spasms responsible for symptoms. This is extremely useful in many different disorders, all of which have in common some element of muscle overactivity. Even when pain is not the overriding complaint, neutralizing facial muscles in this way can make you look younger and feel better.

HERE'S WHAT'S NEW • New applications for Botox are being reported almost daily. It is effective in patients with an overactive bladder (see page 203) and is being used to treat stuttering, facial tics, carpal tunnel syndrome, and tennis elbow. Other uses include the following:

Prostate enlargement. Italian researchers injected Botox directly into an enlarged prostate gland and reduced the frequency of nighttime awakenings to empty the bladder.

Migraine headache. More than half the patients who suffer from migraines experience relief when Botox is injected into the muscles in the forehead, side of the head, back of the head near the neck, the eye, or the brow area. It paralyzes and relaxes the spasm responsible for the pain.

Crossed eyes or lazy eye (strabismus). When the overactive muscles that cause crossed eyes are paralyzed by tiny doses of botulinum toxin, the remaining muscles function properly so that the patient's vision is corrected. The FDA approved Botox for this purpose back in 1989.

Excessive sweating (hyperhidrosis). When injected into any part of the body such as the armpits or hands, Botox can block the chemical transmitter that causes sweating.

Anal fissures. Cracks in the skin around the anus are vulnerable to infection and pain. Injecting Botox into the area reduces the action of the anal sphincter that controls nearby muscles responsible for the cracking. Such injections can be as effective as surgery.

Eye twitching (blepharospasm). A small amount of the toxin injected into the offending muscle relieves the twitching. This beneficial effect was first noted in patients who were given Botox for their wrinkles.

Cerebral palsy. When Botox is injected into spastic or stiff muscles of individuals with cerebral palsy, their symptoms improve sufficiently to permit the use of physical therapy to stretch their muscles and stimulate normal growth.

Cervical dystonia. In this painful condition, muscles in the neck and shoulders cramp so severely that they cause an abnormal positioning of the head. Injecting the involved muscles with Botox relieves the spasm. The FDA approved Botox for this purpose in December 2000.

Stroke. Many stroke victims develop spasms that leave their muscles rigid and cause them to clench their hands. Botox relaxes these muscles, making it possible for them to use their hands and arms again.

Temporomandibular joint disorder (TMJ). Botox has been successfully used to relieve the symptoms of TMJ since 1998. Injected into the muscles of the area, it relieves some of the spasm and improves pain in the jaw joint.

Severe gastroesophageal reflux disease (GERD). When all else has failed, some doctors inject the sphincter between the food pipe and the upper stomach with Botox. This sometimes relieves the spasm of the muscles in the area that cause regurgitation of food and acid responsible for the symptoms of this disorder.

Vocal cord spasm. The most recent use of Botox is its injection into the vocal cords to improve voice quality in a condition called adductor spasmodic dysphonia (AdSD), in which the muscles that control the vocal cords go into spasm. Local injections of Botox every 6 months can relieve these symptoms.

Vocal cord injections of Botox are also being used for "cosmetic" purposes. People whose careers or livelihood depend on the quality of their voices are flocking to specialists for these injections to restore vocal timbre that has been affected by the aging process.

Side effects from Botox are relatively minor. They include respiratory infection, nausea, temporary eyelid droop, and headache. One drawback of Botox injections anywhere is that they almost always have to be repeated every few weeks or months—and they're not cheap. And, of course, there is also the fear that the body's immune system will one day reject Botox. However, to date there has not been evidence of this.

THE BOTTOM LINE • Botox has been around for about 20 years. Its uses and indications continue to multiply. Beyond its cosmetic benefits, injection of Botox continues to have important medical uses.

OVERWEIGHT

_{· · · · · · · · ·}

Does Liposuction Really Help?

OBESITY. OVERWEIGHT. Call it what you will. If you're fat, you're in trouble. Our main concern used to be cosmetic, to look as attractive and young as possible. Those are still goals for most people, but now we have also come to realize that extra fat is a threat to our health. In a real and measurable way, being overweight predisposes us to diabetes (with all its complications), premature heart attack and stroke, and even cancer. So many of us diet for a combination of reasons. Some of us diet with success, but according to the statistics, most usually do not.

We Americans are constantly looking for the quick fix, whether it's feasting on vitamins to make up for not eating properly, or taking "happy pills" to feel good without bothering to figure out what is stressing us, or popping "pep" pills to stay awake during the day after shortchanging ourselves in the sleep department. Along those lines, liposuction is a quick way to eliminate lots of fat, trim your waistline, and look a whole lot better. Liposuction is currently the most popular form of cosmetic surgery in the United States, with almost 400,000 procedures performed every year.

HERE'S WHAT'S NEW

Although liposuction improves your looks, it won't improve your health. According to the latest research, it's not how much fat you remove but *how you do it* that counts. Doctors at Washington University School of Medicine in St. Louis checked the blood chemistry and blood pressure in 15 obese women before they underwent cosmetic liposuction, and again 3 months later. The liposuction left them all looking significantly slimmer, but their medical and biochemical profiles were exactly the same as when they were "fat."

There are several reasons for this lack of measurable benefit after all that fat was removed. For example, it may be that reevaluating these patients 3 months after their surgery is too soon, and that some improvement might become apparent 6 months or 1 year later. It's also possible that this procedure leaves too much body fat behind, or perhaps the deeper fat not accessible to liposuction is the dangerous kind, rather than that which is superficially located and surgically removable. It may also be that the fat cells must shrink in size, not just in number (dieting does make fat cells smaller to improve one's health), or the body needs to run an energy deficit through diet and exercise in order to result in a better body chemistry profile. Whatever the reason, simply eliminating the fat tissue by liposuction doesn't really reduce vulnerability to disease, at least over the short term.

THE BOTTOM LINE

Almost 400,000 men and women undergo liposuction every year to remove excess body fat from their bellies, buttocks, or wherever it happens to be deposited. This improves their looks, their self-image, and even their weight. Unfortunately, however, it does not correct the abnormal chemical profile associated with obesity that predisposes to other diseases. Diet and exercise remain the most effective ways to do so.

Low-Carb Diets—A Change of Heart?

THERE IS NO QUESTION that Robert Atkins, M.D., revolutionized the way Americans eat. His carte blanche diet permitting unlimited consumption of virtually any greasy, fatty food, along with his condemnation of carbs (did you ever dream that McDonald's and Burger King would one day sell hamburgers without buns?), has helped the Mad Cow–beleaguered beef industry and at the same time has hurt bread and pasta makers. In last year's edition of *Breakthrough Health,* I noted that the Atkins regimen has been anathema to the American Heart Association (AHA) and the cardiology community because it flies in the face of all the accumulated data showing that diets rich in saturated fats and cholesterol contribute to heart attacks and strokes.

However, until his untimely death in April 2003, Dr. Atkins continued steadfastly to insist that his diet neither raises cholesterol nor causes arteriosclerosis. He asserted that eating all the butter, cream, fatty meat, and bacon that your heart desires actually *improves* the fat profile of the blood.

HERE'S WHAT'S NEW

According to a representative of the Atkins company, Dr. Atkins's main focus has always been the low-carbohydrate aspect of his diet, and he preferred that only 20 percent of calories come from saturated fat. This executive says, "Not making a distinction between one kind of protein and another was a mistake, and that is why we had to write another book, to get the story straight."

The Atkins group continues to emphasize the low-carb diet and permits unlimited consumption of *unsaturated* fat—with which no one argues. This means more fat from vegetable oils and fish—and less from meat, cheese, and butter.

There have been two more illuminating studies of the safety and effectiveness of a low-carbohydrate diet. One of them was done at Duke University in Durham, North Carolina; the other, at the VA Medical Center in Philadelphia. Although their findings were similar, their conclusions and recommendations differed.

Both the Duke and the VA studies showed that dieters on low-carbohydrate plans do not necessarily enjoy better health benefits over the long term than do those who follow the AHA-recommended low-saturated-fat diet. Although the low-carb group in the VA study lost an average of 13 pounds after 6 months, as compared with only 4 pounds in the low-fat group, the difference between the two after 12 months was not statistically significant (11 pounds for the low-carb and 8 pounds for the low-fat). Interestingly, the low-carb and low-fat dieters in both the VA and the Duke studies had "fairly high" dropout rates, meaning that most people were not prepared to follow either of these diets for any length of time. However, in both studies, the low-carb eaters had a decrease in their triglyceride levels—so that regimen was touted as being cardioprotective and a boon to people with diabetes, in whom, according to results of the VA study, blood sugars were better controlled. In the Duke study, those who lost weight in both the low-carb and low-fat groups enjoyed an overall lower cholesterol level (as is usually the result of weight loss due to any cause).

You'd think that would be enough to recommend a low-carb diet to anyone who can and will follow it. Not as far as the Physicians Committee for Responsible Medicine is concerned. Its spokespersons have urged the Secretary of the Department of Health and Human Services to "convene a panel to investigate the potential adverse effects of low-carbohydrate diets on cholesterol levels, as well as on calcium losses" (the latter effect being another consequence of low-carb diets).

These physicians are worried about the fact that in the Duke study "bad" (LDL) cholesterol levels rose significantly in 30 percent of the 45 low-carb dieters—one from 182 to 219 in 4 weeks, another from 184 to 283 in 12 weeks. (Recommended levels are below 100.) The physicians fear that, despite all the other findings, an LDL rise of this magnitude in one-third of low-carb dieters poses a significant threat.

THE BOTTOM LINE

In all fairness to Dr. Atkins and the heirs of his theory, I am not jumping on the I-told-you-so bandwagon. The fundamental principle behind the Atkins diet has not really changed; it still permits twice as much saturated fat as does the AHA. Dr. Atkins's main recommendation all along was low carbohydrate intake. In his view, whatever else you eat is incidental. Successors to Atkins have emphasized that point, but possibly to escape the wrath of the AHA, they have cautioned about consuming too much saturated fat.

The main downside to limiting fruit and vegetable intake in a low-carb diet is that these foods protect against heart disease and cancer. If you choose to restrict them, I suggest that you take a multivitamin/mineral supplement (although food in its natural form is the best source). As far as saturated fat is concerned, don't have all you want, as Dr. Atkins himself once advised. Focus instead on the polyunsaturated and monounsaturated fats found in vegetable oils and fish.

What this diet debate boils down to is what many doctors have been telling their patients for years. In most cases, weight control reflects a balance between calories in and calories out, with exercise as important an arbiter as any dietary modification. Having said that, the bottom line I suggest to my own patients is that, yes, they should limit carbohydrates, notably white bread, pasta, potatoes, and concentrated sweets. At the same time, they should decrease their intake of foods containing saturated fats and trans fatty acids, such as dairy products and visible fat on meat. And do lots of exercise regularly.

PARKINSON'S DISEASE

The Inflammation Connection

PARKINSON'S DISEASE is an incurable, progressive disorder of the central nervous system that affects at least 500,000 people in the United States with 50,000 new cases reported every year. The disease comes on gradually, and its main symptoms are a resting hand tremor (one that disappears or lessens when you reach for something); rigidity of the arms and legs; overall slowing of body movements; loss of balance; and difficulty walking. It's easy to recognize people with the full-blown condition: They walk with a shuffle, stoop forward, and often have a blank expression. However, there is a spectrum of severity, so the disease is barely apparent in some and all too obvious in others.

Parkinson's usually affects people in their late fifties or early sixties, although it can strike in the forties or even earlier (as was the case with Michael J. Fox). This disease results from the loss of cells in a part of the brain called the substantia nigra. These cells make dopamine, a chemical messenger that transmits signals throughout the brain. Dopamine deficiency causes critical nerve cells in the brain (neurons) to fire haphazardly, leaving those afflicted unable to control their movements.

Although there is no cure for Parkinson's, many drugs can improve its symptoms. The most effective one is levodopa (Larodopa), whose long-term use may unfortunately cause additional significant movement disorders. There are also dopamine agonists that stimulate dopamine receptors in the brain so that patients are able to function a little better with what little dopamine they have. Other medications include Carbex (selegiline), Symmetrel (amantadine), and various anticholinergic agents (the latter should be used with caution in the elderly).

The most recent additions to the anti-Parkinson's armamentarium are the COMT inhibitors. They enhance the effects of levodopa but have potentially serious side effects. There are also several medical and surgical therapies, such as globus pallidus internal-segment pallidotomy and deep brain stimulation. A highly controversial yet promising technique is transplantation with fetal cells to replace the missing ones that make dopamine. This therapy is currently in clinical trials. Researchers have also been conducting studies on using large doses of coenzyme Q_{10} (CoQ_{10}) to treat early Parkinson's disease (see page 218).

HERE'S WHAT'S NEW

Researchers at the Harvard School of Public Health have been periodically reevaluating some 44,000 men and almost 100,000 women over the last 14 years with respect to many diseases, 415 of whom developed Parkinson's disease. The scientists conducting these studies wanted to know how those who came down with Parkinson's differed from those who didn't. They discovered that men and women who had used aspirin or other nonsteroidal anti-inflammatory drugs (NSAIDs) at least twice a day were 45 percent less likely to be diagnosed with Parkinson's disease than those who didn't take medications or did so less frequently. Animal studies had previously suggested that NSAIDs may protect against Parkinson's disease and even Alzheimer's, but this study is the first to show the link in so large a number of men and women.

Although the researchers feel that it's premature to recommend at this time that we should take these drugs to reduce the risk of Parkinson's, they believe that future research will confirm and further clarify their results. It remains to be determined which NSAIDs are most protective and at what dose, the extent of the protection, and whether they might delay the progression of Parkinson's in those who already have it.

It may be years before definitive results are obtained. Since, however, there are so many other reasons for older adults to take aspirin anyway—for example, if you are at high risk for heart attacks and strokes or you have already been stricken—it seems like a good idea for anyone with a family history of Parkinson's disease to take a 325-milligram aspirin tablet a day. Remember, though, that long-term use of NSAIDs and aspirin can result in gastrointestinal bleeding. If you're taking them, be sure to be monitored for this complication.

THE BOTTOM LINE

Parkinson's disease is a progressive neurological disorder for which there is no prevention or cure. However, there are many medications that can help control the symptoms. Gene therapy and stem cell replacement hold promise in the future. Results of a long-term study on many thousands of men and women suggest that taking aspirin or an NSAID on a regular basis can reduce the risk of developing

Parkinson's disease by nearly half. Although these observations are preliminary, it seems like a good idea for anyone who is at a particular risk for Parkinson's disease by virtue of a strong family history to begin such prophylactic therapy, especially since these drugs are relatively safe and widely used anyway. The major complication to look out for with their ongoing use is the risk of gastrointestinal bleeding.

CoQ$_{10}$—The Good and the Bad

COENZYME Q$_{10}$ (COQ$_{10}$) IS A NATURAL ENZYME made in the body and used by its cells to produce the energy they need to continue to function and grow. It is also an antioxidant that protects against free radicals—the waste products of metabolism that can damage vital cellular processes. The heart, liver, kidneys, and pancreas contain the largest amounts of CoQ$_{10}$, the levels of which decrease as we get older.

Do CoQ$_{10}$ supplements prevent or modify disease in any way? According to several small studies and many unsubstantiated anecdotal reports, CoQ$_{10}$ is great for whatever ails you—it improves cardiac function, protects against cancer, helps patients with AIDS, prevents migraine, lowers cholesterol levels, and does countless other wonderful things, all without serious side effects. Little, if any, of this has been confirmed by the medical establishment in large-scale formal scientific evaluations. Nevertheless, CoQ$_{10}$ continues to be very widely used and entices many people. I never took it seriously myself until I read the following.

HERE'S WHAT'S NEW

Neuroscientists at the University of California, San Diego, conducted a study of 80 patients with mild Parkinson's disease who did not as yet require any treatment. This research was done with the usual double-blind method, giving half of the subjects a placebo and the others large doses of CoQ_{10} (1,200 milligrams a day instead of the usual 5 to 200 milligrams). Sixteen months later, those who had taken the CoQ_{10} showed less of the expected progression of their disease than did the placebo-treated group. The researchers emphasize that more studies are needed to confirm these findings.

Neurologists at my own medical center (Weill-Cornell in New York City) were so impressed with these preliminary findings that they have launched a large study, currently in progress. I'm sure other institutions are also testing this supplement in their patients with early, mild Parkinson's disease.

In yet another and different problem area, researchers reported in the journal *Fertility and Sterility* that 22 infertile men who had lower-than-usual levels of CoQ_{10} in their seminal fluid had better sperm motility after taking 200 milligrams of CoQ_{10} daily for 6 months— again, without apparent side effects. This benefit is presumed to be due to the antioxidant effect of the CoQ_{10} on the testes.

This all sounds very good; however, there is a major downside to the CoQ_{10} story. As I reported in the 2004 edition of *Breakthrough Health,* several herbal supplements, including echinacea, do not contain the ingredients listed on their labels. This apparently is also true for CoQ_{10}. ConsumerLab.com, an independent testing company, reviewed 32 different CoQ_{10} products currently on the market and found that several did not contain what their labels said they did. They had either much less that the claimed amount (one product had only 71 percent) or too much (175 percent). These discrepancies are the result of the FDA not overseeing the manufacturing and labeling of these supplements because they are classified as foods, not drugs.

THE BOTTOM LINE

Keep your eye on CoQ_{10}. There may be some good things in the offing. If you have early Parkinson's, ask your doctor about joining one of the several CoQ$_{10}$ studies now being carried out. You may even want to consider taking it independently but under your doctor's supervision. Also, if you're male and infertile, there's no harm in taking 200 milligrams a day. It may give your sperm a needed boost. If you do decide to take CoQ$_{10}$, you may want to check www.ConsumerLab.com for a list of the companies whose products did contain the claimed amount of CoQ$_{10}$.

What the Doctor Ordered?

COFFEE BENEFITS Over the years, there has been no evidence in human studies that coffee has any effect, one way or another, on the development or subsequent course of Parkinson's disease.

HERE'S WHAT'S NEW • A recently completed study of 8,000 Japanese American men living in Hawaii found that the more coffee they drank, the smaller their risk of developing Parkinson's disease. Those who took between 3 and 5 cups a day had a 20 percent lower incidence than those who drank none. Preliminary findings from Massachusetts General Hospital in Boston suggest that, at least in mice, coffee prevents the depletion of dopamine from the brain cells. (Dopamine deficiency is responsible for the symptoms of Parkinson's disease.)

THE BOTTOM LINE • Although it would seem logical that coffee might aggravate some symptoms of Parkinson's disease, especially the tremor, this is not substantiated by any clinical observations. Coffee appears to be good for anyone with Parkinson's, and what's more, drinking it regularly may reduce your risk of ever developing it.

PREGNANCY AND CHILDBIRTH

· · · · · · · · ·

What's Good (and What's Not) When You're Pregnant

PREGNANT WOMEN ARE GIVEN a long list of do's and don'ts to follow for those 9 months they are with child. The first "do" is to find a good obstetrician and have him or her monitor your progress closely until you give birth. That's the easy part. The rest of the advice is not always so easy—or fun.

For example, for the duration of your pregnancy, you will have to give up things that you enjoy—some permanently, such as tobacco (you don't want to expose your infant to secondhand smoke that you're inhaling) and alcohol (even an occasional drink is forbidden). If you faithfully act on all this advice, you can expect to give birth to a healthy, bouncing baby. Here's a quick review of the basics.

Don't . . .

- Drink alcohol—no beer, wine, or hard liquor.

- Take any drugs that were not prescribed by your doctor. That includes herbs, vitamins, and over-the-counter medications. Tell any health-care practitioner you're seeing that you're pregnant. He or she may not know, and it may not be obvious early on.

- Smoke. If you do, you may give birth to your baby too early, it may be underweight, and it could be vulnerable to serious medical problems.

- Have unprotected sex. Pregnancy increases the risk of sexually transmitted diseases, especially HIV/AIDS.

- Use saunas and hot tubs. Excessive heat can hurt the baby.

- Have any medical x-rays.

- Clean or change the kitty litter. Cat's waste may contain a parasite that can hurt your baby.

The list of basics that pregnant women *should* do is almost as daunting.

Do . . .

- Eat at least three regular meals a day or six small ones.

- Exercise regularly.

- Brush and floss your teeth at least once a day and see your dentist regularly.

- Take folic acid supplements every day to prevent spina bifida (a birth defect resulting in abnormal development of the lower spinal cord).

- Take iron and calcium supplements or eat lots of foods that are rich in these minerals.

- Check the directions and warnings on any paint, cleaner, bug spray, or any other chemical with which you come in contact.

Despite adhering to these do's and don'ts, many women experience morning sickness. In fact, more than 80 percent of pregnant women suffer from it during the early stages of pregnancy. Aside from the recurrent nausea and vomiting, they are also likely to experience dizziness, light-headedness, and unusual fatigue. Harvard researchers have found that the incidence of morning sickness is highest among those women who eat lots of saturated fat, mainly meat and dairy products. They may also be sensitive to certain odors and foods.

Eating small amounts of a particular food may relieve the symptoms. You'll have to discover which one(s) help you, since the response varies from woman to woman. Drink lots of fluids, too, and eat whatever you can tolerate when symptoms of morning sickness peak. Dry crackers are especially well tolerated.

Several over-the-counter drugs, such as Dramamine, Benadryl, and Bonine, are widely used to control the nausea and vomiting, although the FDA has not approved any for this purpose. Supplemental vitamin B_6 (10 to 25 milligrams three times a day), as well as 5 milligrams of vitamin K and/or 25 milligrams of vitamin C, also has been reported to help. Some doctors have found that large doses of adrenal cortical extract can stop the nausea and vomiting, but this therapy may be risky.

Over the centuries, there have been anecdotal reports, mainly from China and India, that ginger alleviates the symptoms of morning sickness. Acupuncture and acupressure have their proponents, too.

HERE'S WHAT'S NEW

There is no way to hide from the pregnancy police—the list of do's and don'ts keeps getting longer. The good news first. Scientists at the University of Helsinki in Finland have found that children born to women who ate chocolate while pregnant have a happier disposition; they laugh and smile more than do those whose mothers had no chocolate. What's more, if a woman was especially stressed during her pregnancy and ate chocolate, her baby showed less fear of new situations. The researchers are not sure what chemicals in the chocolate are responsible for this positive effect, but who cares if you like chocolate?

Chocolate may be good for your baby, but there's no evidence that it reduces morning sickness. That's where ginger comes in. Although this herb is widely promoted to minimize motion sickness, women have been hesitant to use it for morning sickness because it contains compounds that have been shown to cause chromosomal changes in the test tube. Recent studies indicate, however, that small amounts of ginger are safe and effective. Take it in divided doses (250 milligrams three times a day after meals and one at bedtime), but no more than 1 gram (or four tablets) a day. Vitamin B_6 in a dose of 25 milligrams three times a day is as effective as ginger, equally safe, and without major side effects, either to the mother or the fetus.

An estimated 10 to 16 percent of pregnant women suffer from depression. The FDA has expressed concern about treating them with antidepressant drugs, including the Prozac family of selective serotonin reuptake inhibitors (SSRIs) as well as others. This has been the case especially in the last trimester because newborns may experience jitters, tremors, breathing problems, difficulty sleeping, and other withdrawal symptoms. Although these usually clear up in a few days, they can last longer. Antidepressants not only are potentially harmful to the fetus, they increase the risk of premature delivery. It's important for depressed pregnant women to be treated, because serious depression can cause malnutrition that can harm the baby, or lead to suicide. Discuss with your doctor whether the benefits of your taking an antidepressant outweigh the risks. It's important for you both to determine which medication is best for your needs, in what dose, and for how long. One option to consider is to taper the drugs 10 to 14 days before your due date.

Most women (and doctors) know better than to permit chest x-rays to be done during pregnancy, but they may not give as much thought to dental x-rays. Researchers at the University of Washington in Seattle have found conclusive evidence in a large survey of pregnant women that having dental x-rays is more likely to lead to the birth of an infant who weighs less than normal. This had previously been shown for medical x-rays but not for dental radiation.

If you suffer from epilepsy, remember that uncontrolled seizures during pregnancy can cause a miscarriage. There are many antiseizure drugs available, but some are safer than others. Researchers at Emory University in Atlanta recently reported that children born to women who use Depakote (divalproex) are more likely to have birth defects and other problems. A Vancouver study reported that 11 percent of children born of mothers taking Depakote had birth defects, mostly spina bifida (in which the development of the spinal cord is incomplete). Folic acid is taken routinely by pregnant women to prevent spina bifida, but women taking Depakote may need 10 times the usual dosage. The Emory researchers recommend avoiding this drug not only during pregnancy but also during the childbearing years. They also report that the newer antiseizure medication Lamictal (lamotrigine), though safer than Depakote, still affects 2 percent of children of mothers who took it.

Researchers at the University of Texas Southwestern Medical Center in Dallas recently tested more than 17,000 women receiving prenatal medical care. They did routine blood tests on all of them to measure their thyroid function, regardless of whether or not they had any symptoms of thyroid malfunction.

Most doctors do not routinely check the thyroid in pregnant women unless they have reason to do so. In the course of this routine blood test, these investigators found 404 women who had no idea that their thyroid gland was underactive, or hypothyroid. (Hypothyroidism classically leaves you tired, sensitive to cold, a little constipated, with a tendency to gain weight or have trouble losing it, and dry skin. These are such common symptoms that they are often ignored.)

There were twice as many premature births in this group than in those with normal thyroid function. Another study in 1999 had found that mothers with untreated hypothyroidism in pregnancy, regardless of whether it caused any symptoms, were more likely to give birth to children with lowered IQs. That's because thyroid hormones are important for brain development, and in the first 3 months, the fetus is entirely dependent on the mother to provide them.

Despite these findings, there is some disagreement about whether every pregnant woman should have her thyroid function tested (it is not done routinely in the United States). The only possible reason not to that I can think of is cost. However, the British government, obviously suspecting that it may be more economical to do so, is now in the process of deciding whether such testing should be mandatory.

In the meantime, everyone agrees that (a) women who are known to be hypothyroid should be retested during pregnancy to make sure they are taking enough of the thyroid supplement, and (b) since pregnant and nursing women need 220 to 290 micrograms of iodine a day (as compared with the 150 micrograms that other adults require), prenatal vitamins should contain iodine, essential for normal thyroid function. Check the label on your multivitamin bottle; one-third of them do not have iodine.

THE BOTTOM LINE

These findings create more fodder—both good and bad—for the pregnancy police. Chocolate benefits children whose mothers eat it while pregnant. Ginger and vitamin B₆ are safe and effective against morning sickness. Avoid dental x-rays because the radiation exposure is considered just as dangerous as medical x-rays. If you're taking an antidepressant like Prozac (fluoxetine), don't stop it before discussing it with your doctor. Being depressed while you're pregnant can harm you, and you must balance the positive and negative effects of this drug. If you are epileptic, it's important to take antiseizure medication. The one to avoid is Depakote; the safest appears to be the newer Lamictal, although it too may occasionally cause problems for the fetus.

A routine blood test to screen for thyroid function is not expensive. Since an underfunctioning gland may not produce recognizable symptoms but can have serious consequences, I advise all my pregnant patients to get a thyroid test.

Beware of Mercury in Fish

EVERYONE KNOWS THAT FISH is probably the healthiest food we can eat. A single 4-ounce serving provides between 30 and 50 percent of our daily protein requirement and contains all the essential amino acids we need. Fish liver oil is an exceptional source of vitamins A and D. Minerals such as phosphorus, copper, iron, calcium, and iodine are especially abundant in salt-water fish and are necessary for everything from aiding growth and tissue repair to composition of bone, digestive juices, and cellular fluids. The omega-3 polyunsaturated fats in fish maintain skin health, normal liver and kidney function, and lower cholesterol levels. They also minimize the number of asthmatic attacks, improve mood, and render the blood less likely to clot. For all these and many other reasons, fish eaters have fewer heart attacks and strokes.

Unfortunately, the mercury content of some fish presents a potential problem to pregnant women and nursing mothers—yet another "don't." In the 2004 edition of *Breakthrough Health,* I reported that there are many different types of mercury and some that contaminate fish might not be harmful. I haven't seen any further reports on this theory and can only assume that it has not been substantiated. What then should pregnant women do about eating fish?

HERE'S WHAT'S NEW

The FDA has now officially warned pregnant women, nursing mothers, and women who may become pregnant not to eat fish with high mercury content—notably shark, swordfish, king mackerel, and tilefish—and to limit their intake of a variety of other fish and shellfish that are lower in mercury (including canned tuna) to 12 ounces, or two average meals a week. Mercury levels in tuna can vary. Fresh tuna steaks have more than canned light tuna. So eat no more than 6 ounces (one average meal) of albacore tuna (tuna steaks or canned white tuna) a week. The same restrictions apply to young children.

If you eat fresh fish from neighborhood lakes, rivers, and coastal areas, check local advisories about whether it's safe to consume them. If that information is not available, limit your intake to 6 ounces per week and don't have any other fish that week.

Why the fear of mercury? A recent report from the Environmental Protection Agency estimates that 630,000 children were born between 1999 and 2000 with blood mercury levels higher than the 5.8 parts per billion established as the upper limit of safety. Furthermore, researchers at the Harvard School of Public Health have shown that children exposed to mercury while still in the womb may suffer permanent damage to their hearts and brains.

How much fish should women (and men) beyond childbearing age eat? The general recommendation is at least two servings a week (a serving being defined as 140 grams). At least one of these should be oily fish—salmon, herring (the oiliest of all), mackerel, sardines, tuna, and others. Oily fish contain the beneficial omega-3 fatty acids (see pages 80 and 137). Canned tuna doesn't count as oily because the canning process reduces the omega-3 fatty acid content so that it's comparable to that of nonoily fish. You should probably not eat more than four portions of *any* fish per week because of the risk of contamination by dioxin and PCB, common industrial contaminants.

THE BOTTOM LINE

To avoid the possibility of mercury contamination, pregnant women, nursing mothers, young children, and women of childbearing age should limit their intake of fish to 12 ounces a week, of which no more than 6 ounces should be albacore tuna. But everyone should have at least one serving per week of an oily fish, such as salmon and mackerel, for the benefit their omega-3 fatty acid content confers on the cardiovascular system. Pregnant women need them as well (but no more than one serving a week) in order to ensure normal brain development of the fetus. If you can't or won't eat fish, then take at least 1 gram a day of the omega-3 capsule supplements. They do not contain significant amounts of mercury.

WHAT THE DOCTOR ORDERED?

CUT BACK ON COFFEE Heavy coffee consumption is often accompanied by use of tobacco or alcohol. That may be in part why doctors have always had reservations about pregnant women drinking coffee during pregnancy. Most still recommend a limit of 300 milligrams of caffeine at day during the 9 months of pregnancy. Since there are 80 to 130 milligrams per cup of coffee, depending on its size (an 8-ounce cup has about 85 milligrams), this essentially means no more than 3 cups a day.

HERE'S WHAT'S NEW • The body metabolizes caffeine more slowly during pregnancy, especially during the last few months. Some of the old wives' tales about coffee and pregnancy have turned out to be fairly accurate; others have not. A recent research review concluded that pregnant women who drink an average of 2 cups of coffee a day are at 1.4 times greater risk of miscarriage than those who consume less than that. In another study, however, it took 6 cups to increase the likelihood of a miscarriage or still-birth. Consuming 8 or more cups a day increased the risk of still-births by 220 percent compared with women who drank 4 to 7 cups a day, and by 300 percent compared with women who did not drink coffee at all! The ingredient in the brew responsible for this problem has not been identified.

There is some evidence that coffee boosts male fertility. Brazilian researchers from São Paulo University found that men who drink 1 to 3 cups of coffee per day produce sperm that are more motile, which could improve the chances of pregnancy.

THE BOTTOM LINE • Although the numbers vary, there is a consensus that coffee drinking should be reduced during the 9 months of pregnancy. Many doctors believe that up to 300 milligrams of caffeine (about 3 cups of coffee) is a safe upper limit for pregnant women. Others recommend no more than 2 cups a day. Complications of excessive coffee intake include not only miscarriage and stillbirth but also preterm birth and low birth weight. Fetal abnormalities are not believed to be a consequence.

The same advice about caffeine consumption during pregnancy also applies to the breastfeeding period, since caffeine enters breast milk and can cause the baby to become jittery. So it boils down to this: The less coffee you drink when you're pregnant or nursing, the better.

Avoid Ginseng during Pregnancy

GINSENG HAS BEEN VALUED as a medicine in China for more than 2000 years. It was once held in such high regard that only the emperor was allowed to grow it. It continues to be used by many Asians as well as millions the world over, including Americans, to boost physical and mental vitality. A report in 2001 claimed that more than 9 percent of pregnant women worldwide use herbal supplements and up to 10 percent of those in Asia take ginseng during pregnancy. How many do so in this country has not yet been determined, but the sales of ginseng are in the many millions of dollars annually. You can take this herb as a capsule, tablet, tea, tincture, powder, or extract, and it is also added to cosmetics, candies, and soft drinks. (I don't happen to like its taste.)

Several different types of ginseng currently are cultivated around the world. The major ones belong to the Panax family, one species of which is grown in Asia and another in North America. The words *Panax* and *panacea* are both derived from the Greek term for "all-healing," probably stemming from the ancient (and to a great extent, modern) belief that ginseng is indeed a miracle herb.

Ginseng's greatest scientific endorsement is to be found in the Chinese and Russian medical literature. To the best of my knowledge, there have been few studies in this country that have verified the European and Asian observations that ginseng improves athletic performance, enhances physical and mental ability, prevents stress ulcers, fights inflammation and cancer, and lowers cholesterol and triglyceride levels. Some gynecologists have published accounts of its effectiveness in treating the hot flashes of menopausal women. If ginseng does so, then it's probably because of its estrogen-like compounds, in which event I would be as cautious about women using it as I am about black cohosh (see page 51).

The major active ingredients actually identified in ginseng are steroidlike substances called ginsenosides. Ginseng enthusiasts call them adaptogens and claim they stimulate the immune system and possess antistress properties—a concept I find rather vague.

Since there's no standardized international method for extracting ginsenosides from the herb, it's almost impossible to interpret any of the existing research data about its effectiveness or to decide what doses to use for treating any disorder. To make matters worse, analyses of ginseng products purchased by mail order or at health food stores revealed that some samples contained few active ginsenosides, while others had many more than was claimed. They differed so much in potency that it's difficult, if not impossible, to decide how much to take of any given brand. (This is also true for several other popular herbs.) Then there is also the question of adulteration. Given the lack of supervision by the FDA over the production methods for ginseng and other herbs and "nutritional supplements," it's not surprising that batches of ginseng have been found to be contaminated by a variety of toxins.

Ginseng is known to elevate blood pressure and cause insomnia, diarrhea, skin rashes, vaginal bleeding, and painful breasts. (The latter two side effects are probably due to its hormonelike action.) It also thins the blood, so it should not be taken along with anticoagulants such as Coumadin (warfarin) or with nonsteroidal anti-inflammatory drugs. Men and women with diabetes should also be cautious about using ginseng, because when combined with insulin or other diabetic drugs, it can cause an excessive drop in the blood sugar level. There are also reports of headache, tremors, and mania when ginseng is taken along with the antidepressant drug Nardil (phenelzine). Ginseng also may interfere with the action of diuretics.

HERE'S WHAT'S NEW

Researchers at the Chinese University of Hong Kong, Prince of Wales Hospital, have found that one of type of ginsenoside in the herb can cause abnormalities in rat embryos. The researchers worry that ginseng could also have as-yet-unknown harmful effects in human babies, too. For that reason, it seems to me that this herb should not be taken during the first 3 months of pregnancy. Pregnant women should always consult a doctor before taking any herbal supplement.

THE BOTTOM LINE

Although the observations regarding the potential danger of ginseng during pregnancy were made in rats, remember that many other findings in medicine are derived from animal models. In fact, most drugs in development are first tested in animals, many of which often respond very much like we do. Given these suspicious findings, there is no reason for pregnant women to take ginseng since it's certainly not vital, unlike insulin or digitalis or antibiotics. You can safely postpone taking it until after your baby is born and you have finished breastfeeding.

Preventing Stillbirths

STILLBIRTHS OCCUR IN AN ESTIMATED 1 in 200 pregnancies in this country every year. (A stillbirth is defined as the loss of a pregnancy at 20 weeks or later.) In more than one-third of these cases, it is not clear why these children die in the womb, although it does happen more often in mothers with diabetes and high blood pressure. There is ongoing research to identify other risk factors.

HERE'S WHAT'S NEW

Doctors at the Rosie (no relation to me) Hospital in Cambridge, England, have followed the obstetrical history of 120,000 Scottish women after they'd had one child. Of these, 17,000 were delivered by Cesarean and 103,000 vaginally. For those who had previously delivered by Cesarean, the absolute risk of a stillbirth at or after the 39th week of gestation was 1.1 per 1,000; that number was less than half, 0.5 per 1,000, when the first baby had been delivered vaginally.

The researchers conclude that delivery by Cesarean section in the first pregnancy can increase the risk of an unexplained stillbirth in the second. It may be that scar tissue resulting from the incision in the uterus during a Cesarean section affects the function of the placenta so that the fetus is less adequately nourished. This scar tissue is also more likely to cause a life-threatening rupture of the uterus during a subsequent vaginal delivery than if the women have their next baby by Cesarean, too.

THE BOTTOM LINE

If you intend to have more than one child, think twice before you opt to have your first baby delivered by Cesarean section. Doing so doubles the chance that your next baby will be stillborn if you deliver vaginally. If you do need a Cesarean delivery for medical reasons, by all means have it, but then your next baby should also be born by Cesarean. This reduces the risk of a stillbirth as well as the possibility of uterine rupture.

SLEEP PROBLEMS

· · · · · · · · ·

Treating Excessive Daytime Drowsiness

AMONG THE MOST COMMON COMPLAINTS I hear from patients are "I can't seem to get a good night's sleep" and "I'm so tired that I can barely stay awake during the day." There are many possible reasons both for insomnia and the resulting daytime fatigue, and they are often related.

It's obvious that if you're not sleeping long enough or deeply enough, for any reason, you will feel drowsy the next day. Lack of sleep, however, is only one of many reasons for excessive daytime fatigue. Chronic depression, anxiety, and stress can also leave you feeling tired and unable to function properly during the day. So can a hangover from a sleeping pill as well as medications such as antidepressants, antibiotics, and cardiac drugs. You may be chronically tired too because you have disease of the liver, kidneys, heart, or lungs; anemia; a hidden infection; low thyroid function; or even cancer. So if you're abnormally drowsy during the day and you can't figure out why, tell your doctor about it. Don't get hooked on quick fixes—caffeine, other stimulants such as Ritalin (methylphenidate), or amphetamine and any of its derivatives.

In addition to all the above-mentioned reasons, three specific medical conditions can leave you excessively drowsy during the day— shift-work sleep disorder, sleep apnea, and narcolepsy.

Shift-work sleep disorder. Between 5 and 8 percent of the world's population, including approximately 7 million Americans, work permanent or rotating night shifts. This persistently or recurrently disrupts their sleep/wake schedule, causing either extreme sleepiness or insomnia, headaches, and difficulty concentrating.

Obstructive sleep apnea. This condition prevents at least 12 million Americans from having a good night's sleep. It is almost always caused by obstruction of the airways during sleep—usually because the soft tissues at the back of the throat relax and collapse. Sleep apnea can be recognized when loud snoring is interrupted by cycles of silence, during which breathing stops, followed by the gasp of awakening. These cycles occur hundreds of times during the night and result in a lack of deep, adequate sleep, leaving sufferers exhausted and drowsy the following day. Sleep apnea is also associated with increased risk of cardiovascular disease, glaucoma (see page 111), gastric reflux, and elevated blood pressure.

There are several ways to treat sleep apnea, ranging from removing whatever it is that's obstructing the airways to keeping these airways open with a flow of pressurized air through a nasal tube at night (continuous positive airway pressure, or CPAP).

Narcolepsy. An estimated 1 in 2,000 Americans are afflicted with this lifelong disorder, which leaves them constantly and overwhelmingly sleepy and physically so weak that they can even nod off in the middle of a sentence. They repeatedly experience dreamlike hallucinations and often suffer attacks of paralysis for a few seconds throughout the day (cataplexy). Narcolepsy is believed to be caused by the genetic alteration of certain brain chemicals (orexins) with several functions, one of which is to promote wakefulness.

There is no cure for narcolepsy, and for years the only treatments for its symptoms were stimulants such as amphetamine and its various derivatives. These all lent themselves to abuse, dependency, and occasional psychiatric complications. Then came Ritalin, with fewer side effects but still no panacea.

In 1998, the FDA approved Provigil (modafinil), a new safe, effective, and well-tolerated psychostimulant for the treatment of narcolepsy. It promotes wakefulness by acting on the sleep and wake centers in the brain and the cerebral cortex. Its main advantage is that it does not cause generalized stimulation. Provigil reduces the frequency of narcoleptic attacks and leaves patients feeling awake without the jitters, anxiety, and "hyper" feeling caused by amphetamine. At bedtime, there is no carryover from a daytime dose, so one can still enjoy a good night's sleep.

It was only a matter of time before Provigil would be used "off label"—that is, for purposes other than the narcolepsy for which it was approved. Some doctors prescribed it along with other, necessary medications that made their patients sleepy; for men and women who felt they needed more energy during the day; for shift workers; or for students staying up late to study for exams. It has now reached the point where anyone who simply wants to be the life of the party into the wee hours is taking Provigil. Many doctors, including me, worry about this, fearful that this drug will mask the real cause of their fatigue or drive their bodies into prolonged wakefulness and deprive them of the sleep they need.

HERE'S WHAT'S NEW

The FDA has now approved the use of Provigil for two disorders for which it is being widely used anyway: sleep disorders in shift workers and obstructive sleep apnea.

If you fall into either category, your doctor may now prescribe Provigil to help you stay awake. Make sure, however, that you get the 8 hours of sleep you need. If you're working the night shift, take Provigil 1 hour before you start.

If your sleep apnea is well controlled, you don't need Provigil. But if you wake up sleepy in the morning and are drowsy all day despite therapy, Provigil will help. It's safe, nonaddictive, and it has fewer side effects than other stimulants (its effects include mild-to-moderate headache, nervousness, stuffy nose, dizziness, and occasionally an upset stomach). Take it in the morning before going to work. But remember, don't stop any other sleep apnea therapy.

THE BOTTOM LINE

Millions of people have trouble sleeping for a host of different reasons, and they treat the problem in many different ways, depending on the cause. The FDA has approved the use of Provigil for three common disorders that leave people abnormally sleepy during the day: narcolepsy, shift-work disorder, and obstructive sleep apnea. This drug is safe and keeps you awake during the day without significant side effects.

It's tempting to take this drug just to stay awake when you want to party or if you have some other personal reason. I don't encourage that because, being old-fashioned, I don't believe that we should interfere when nature is signaling us that it's time to sleep. Provigil promotes wakefulness but doesn't replace the need for getting enough sleep.

Less Coffee, More Often

MANY OF US, regardless of what we do all day—whether we're doctors, bus drivers, college students, or housewives—depend on one or more cups of coffee before we leave home in the morning to keep us awake and alert through the day. Research has established that coffee improves alertness, concentration, and job performance. But it does have its downside. Too much can make you nervous, and you're better off not having any at bedtime, because it may very well keep you awake.

H E R E ' S   W H A T ' S   N E W

Researchers at the Sleep Disorders Center at Rush University Medical Center in Chicago have come up with some interesting and useful findings. The stimulation we derive from drinking several mugs of coffee at breakfast wears off as the day goes on, just when the body's appetite for sleep begins to increase. Caffeine blocks these sleep-inducing stimuli. On the basis of their study, the Rush doctors recommend that instead of loading up with coffee in the morning before you leave home, you take 2 ounces at frequent intervals throughout the afternoon just before you begin to feel as if you could use a little nap. Doing so will wake you up. What's more, it won't prevent you from sleeping at night.

T H E   B O T T O M   L I N E

Have that cup or two of java in the morning to get you going. But you should know that its effect will wear off when you need it most in the afternoon. The best way to maintain your alertness later in the day is to have frequent small doses (a couple of ounces) of coffee in the afternoon rather than one big slug in the morning.

STROKE

• • • • • • • • • •

Statins to the Rescue

STROKE IS THE third leading cause of death in this country after heart disease and cancer. More than 600,000 Americans have one every year, and 160,000 die from it (more African Americans than Caucasians). In 2002, stroke caused almost 5.5 million deaths world-wide, according to the World Health Organization.

One dictionary definition of the word *stroke* is "to touch lightly and with affection." That is certainly a misnomer as far as the subject of this chapter is concerned. The stroke I'm referring to is damage to the brain that follows a disruption of its blood supply. In about 80 percent of cases, this happens when blood flow within a brain artery is cut off by the rupture of an atherosclerotic plaque or by a fresh clot that has either formed there or traveled from elsewhere in the body. In 20 percent of cases, a stroke is caused when a cerebral blood vessel bursts and hemorrhages into the brain tissue. A stroke can also result from the obstruction of a carotid artery in the neck, which supplies blood to the brain. If treated early enough, clots can be dissolved or otherwise removed to prevent a stroke from occurring.

Symptoms of a stroke, your chances of surviving it, and the quality of your recovery, depend on the amount of brain tissue damaged, its location, the length of time it was deprived of oxygen, and the bodily functions controlled by the area involved. So a stroke may result in weakness or paralysis of an arm or leg, visual problems, speech impairment, or behavioral changes. If only a small artery was involved, the residual symptoms may be trivial and temporary. When the damaged area is large and critically situated, the result can be permanent, devastating, or fatal.

The best way to protect yourself against a stroke is to control the risk factors that predispose you to it. Traditionally, the most important ones have been elevated cholesterol, tobacco use, high blood pressure, overweight, lack of exercise, and diabetes. Over the years, stroke prevention has focused on normalizing these six areas of vulnerability. It's pretty straightforward. All you need is the motivation, discipline, and willpower to do it.

HERE'S WHAT'S NEW

The debate has always revolved around the definition of what constitutes a high cholesterol reading. Ideal target numbers are continually being reduced (see page 171). It has now been shown, however, that cholesterol-lowering drugs can reduce the number of strokes by a third even in people with "normal" readings. Doctors now recommend that everyone at high risk for stroke (people with diabetes, those with a strong family history of cerebrovascular disease or other genetic vulnerability, or any combination of the above risk factors) should take a statin drug, regardless of the cholesterol level (see page 175). This was concluded from the Heart Protection Study reported in the *Lancet* involving 20,000 patients, many of whom had low cholesterol but were otherwise at high risk for a stroke or had already suffered one. Half were given a cholesterol-lowering drug; the others received a placebo. Within 5 years, those on 40 milligrams a day of simvastatin (Zocor) had one-third fewer strokes and heart attacks than the patients who were taking a placebo.

The scientists involved in the study emphasize that we must rethink our present strategy of administering statin drugs only to those with elevated cholesterol levels.

In a study reported in the *Lancet,* scientists emphasized the importance of treating stroke patients as early as possible to increase the odds of their full recovery. The normal treatment window for administering clot-busting drugs after a stroke is 3 hours. These researchers have found that these drugs help even when taken as long as $4^1/_2$ hours after the onset of the stroke symptoms. They are somewhat less effective but still better than no treatment. The drug used in the study was the readily available tPA, tissue plasminogen activator.

THE BOTTOM LINE

Doctors have long recognized the importance of lowering cholesterol to prevent such vascular complications as heart attack and stroke. Using a statin drug in men and women who are otherwise vulnerable to a stroke for other reasons reduces their risk of having one by about 30 percent.

So if you have a bad family history of stroke, or you have high blood pressure, diabetes, or you are or were a smoker, speak to your doctor now about taking a cholesterol-lowering statin medication, regardless of your cholesterol level. Also, treatment with a clot buster, formerly believed to be effective only within 3 hours after the onset of symptoms, is now believed to work as late as $4^1/_2$ hours after the onset of symptoms.

TENDONITIS

·········

Shocking News for Bad Shoulders

DO YOU NEED HELP getting into your jacket or overcoat? Does it hurt when you close the clasp on the back of your necklace? Does shoulder pain prevent you from throwing a football, playing basketball, or doing anything else that requires raising your arms over your head? (My readers never surrender!)

If so, you probably have a problem with your shoulder's rotator cuff, whose function it is to keep the top of the arm bone (humerus) in the shoulder socket (acromium). Consisting of several muscles, tendons, and ligaments, the rotator cuff is vulnerable to tearing. If severe enough, the tear must be surgically repaired.

There is also a common, painful disorder, called calcific tendonitis, in which calcium forms on the tendons and inflames them, restricting mobility of the shoulder joint. Calcific tendonitis occurs

243

most often after age 40, especially in athletes who perform repetitive, vigorous movements of the shoulder while playing football, water polo, baseball, and basketball. Calcific tendonitis is also more common in people with diabetes, who don't heal quite as well as the rest of us.

There are two main types of shoulder calcification other than that seen in athletes—*degenerative* calcification, which occurs in older people and is caused by the normal wear and tear of the joint over the years, and *reactive* calcification, which develops for some unknown reason in younger adults.

In degenerative calcific tendonitis, blood flow to the muscles and tendons decreases with age. They also grow weaker, begin to fray, and become vulnerable to the deposition of calcium that inflames them.

In reactive calcific tendonitis, calcium temporarily settles in the tendons but is then reabsorbed by the body, and the condition clears up as mysteriously as it began, without the need for any specific therapy. If your shoulder pain persists, you have the degenerative type.

There are a number of ways to deal with chronic degenerative calcific tendonitis. But before you decide on any therapy, have an MRI of the affected shoulder to make sure your pain isn't due to a torn rotator cuff. Once you've confirmed the diagnosis of calcific tendonitis, avoid any movements that aggravate the pain. Have someone help you put on your coat, stop playing baseball, and don't engage in any activity that makes the pain worse.

The pain itself can usually be controlled by analgesics. Start with an over-the-counter nonsteroidal anti-inflammatory (NSAID) such as ibuprofen and proceed to prescription-strength medication as needed. See a physiatrist (don't confuse "physiatrist" with "psychiatrist," the former deals with the body; the latter, with the mind), who can plan a program of physiotherapy for you and advise you about a rehabilitation exercise program. If your symptoms continue to be disabling, a steroid injection into the shoulder joint will provide temporary relief; it does not, however, solve the problem.

If you're still in pain, you'll need surgery, in this case, an arthroscopic procedure done under light anesthesia. The arthroscope is a special TV camera that is inserted into the shoulder joint through a small incision in the skin. It enables the surgeon to see exactly where the calcium deposits are located and how extensive they are. Another incision is then made through which instruments are inserted into the joint to remove these deposits. The area is then rinsed to remove any loose calcium crystals that have been left behind and can cause irritation and inflammation. When it's all done, you can go home the same day. You'll need to wear a sling for a few days after the surgery, apply ice, and perhaps have a few sessions of electrical stimulation to promote healing. You should also have a few weeks of follow-up physiotherapy to do range-of-motion, strengthening, and stretching exercises.

HERE'S WHAT'S NEW

Had I known a few months ago what I am about to report to you, I might well have spared my wife two surgical procedures. Researchers in Munich, Germany, have come up with a treatment for degenerative calcific tendonitis that avoids anesthesia and surgery. (Munich is where sound waves were first used to shatter gallstones and kidney stones.) Doctors there have now developed a technique for directing these shock waves toward the shoulder, causing the calcium deposits to disintegrate.

After this treatment, patients underwent 10 physiotherapy sessions that included exercise mobilization techniques, massage, and manual therapy to maintain good range of motion of the joint. During 6 months of follow-up, 144 patients so treated, who would otherwise have needed surgery or repeated steroid injections, enjoyed an 85 percent success rate. The calcific deposits disappeared completely in 60 percent of cases after 6 months, and in 86 percent after 12 months.

The procedure, called extracorporeal shock-wave therapy (ESWT), takes up to 1 hour per session and can require intravenous painkillers, but not general or even local anesthesia. A second course of this shock-wave therapy is given about 2 weeks later.

Exactly how ESWT works is not clear. It may physically disrupt the calcium deposits or increase the spread of an enzyme that does so; it may stimulate the formation of new blood vessels and a significant increase in blood supply that promotes new bone growth in the area—or any combination of these effects. But the end result, as reported in the *Journal of the American Medical Association,* is the elimination of the calcium deposits and the need for surgery or repeated steroid injections.

THE BOTTOM LINE

If you have shoulder pain from chronic calcific tendonitis, ask your doctor about shock-wave therapy to remove the calcium. This is still a relatively new procedure and not yet universally available. Specialists are still trying to determine the optimum strength of the shock waves. I predict, however, that ESWT will soon be widely used. It's worth asking about and waiting for. It can help you avoid surgery and multiple steroid injections (especially undesirable for people with diabetes in whom they make the blood sugar more difficult to control).

ULCER

· · · · · · · · ·

How to Eradicate *H. Pylori*

FIFTY PERCENT OF THE WORLD'S POPULATION harbor a spiral-shaped bacterium called *Helicobacter pylori* (*H. pylori*) in their stomachs. This bug was considered nothing more than a harmless resident of the upper part of the gut until 1982, when two brilliant Australian doctors insisted and proved that it causes stomach ulcers.

Although *H. pylori* usually gives no symptoms to the great majority of people infected with it, it does cause peptic ulcers (those in the stomach and the first part of the small intestine, known as the duodenum), atrophic gastritis (inflammation of the lining of the stomach) in adults and children, and is responsible for a twofold to sixfold increased risk of stomach cancer. Some doctors believe very strongly that we should all be screened for this bug, regardless of whether we have any gastric symptoms, and if found to have it, receive treatment to eradicate it.

Before we knew all this about *H. pylori*, we thought that peptic ulcers were due to spicy food, acid, stress, and other lifestyle characteristics. The majority of patients were treated over the long term with medications, such as H2 blockers and proton pump inhibitors, that focused on reducing acid production by the stomach. Diet was considered to be very important, too, and psychological counseling was also commonly advised. ("You're making me nervous. You're going to give me an ulcer!") Now that we understand the seminal role of *H. pylori* in the development of such ulcers, every person with this disease is screened for this bug and treated for it if it is present. Many ulcer patients have stopped taking the medications they previously were prescribed and are no longer regarded as nervous ninnies.

There are several ways to look for *H. pylori*. It can be diagnosed by measuring its antibodies in the blood. This blood test is 80 to 95 percent accurate. The bacterium can also be found with a breath test. You're given a drink containing urea that has been labeled with radioactive carbon. The amount of this labeled carbon you then exhale is an indicator of the presence of *H. pylori* in your stomach. This test is 94 to 98 percent accurate. If neither of these procedures convinces your doctor, he or she may suggest an upper endoscopy during which the stomach and duodenum are biopsied.

Once the bug is found, there are currently eight different regimens approved by the FDA to eradicate it. Basically, they all consist of a combination of antibiotics such as Amoxicillin or tetracycline (the latter not to be used in kids under 12), along with Flagyl (metronidazole) or Biaxin (clarithromycin), plus an acid blocker such as Prilosec (omeprazole), and Pepto-Bismol (bismuth subsalicylate) for 7 to 14 days. The longer the therapy is continued, the more effective it is said to be. Several of my patients have found that this combination of drugs taken for the recommended period upsets their stomachs. Some were forced to discontinue it after a few days. They worry that they have not eradicated their *H. pylori*. The following research results should encourage them.

HERE'S WHAT'S NEW

Doctors in Canton, Ohio, studied 160 adult men and women whose average age was 50 years and who had dyspepsia and documented *H. pylori* infection. They were all treated with a conventional combination of drugs—two tablets of Pepto-Bismol four times a day; one tablet of Flagyl four times a day; 2 grams of amoxicillin four times a day; and two tablets of Prevacid (lansoprazole), 30 milligrams once a day. But here's the rub. Half the group received this therapy for the full 7 days; *the other half took it for only 1 day!*

Guess what? When the subjects were restudied 5 weeks later, the bacteria had been eliminated in 95 percent of those who followed the 1-day regimen; the 7-day group had a success rate of only 90 percent!

Frankly, I'm surprised at these results and don't quite know how to explain them. But if it really does work, there are obvious advantages to taking this pile of drugs for only 1 day rather than 7. In addition to the convenience, there is also the matter of cost. I would like to see a follow-up study looking at the recurrence rate in both groups months down the line. In the meantime, I am still suggesting the 7-day course to my patients who can tolerate and afford it. To those who can't, I prescribe the 1-day course described above and follow them closely. If additional studies verify that the 1-day treatment really works and the *H. pylori* doesn't recur, then I will recommend it for everybody.

Austrian researchers have found that, in addition to its effects on the gastrointestinal tract, eradicating an *H. pylori* infection raises the level of the "good" HDL cholesterol and improves the overall lipid profile (cholesterol and all its related fats) in the blood. I'm not suggesting that if you have high cholesterol, you should get yourself tested for *H. pylori* (unless, of course, you also have stomach symptoms). But if you happen to be treated for *H. pylori,* don't be surprised if your cholesterol profile improves.

THE BOTTOM LINE

If you have chronic indigestion, ulcer symptoms, or a documented peptic ulcer, you should be tested for *H. pylori.* You may very well be infected with it. This organism can be eradicated by means of a combination of antibiotics, antibacterials, and acid-reducing drugs. Traditionally, these medications have been prescribed for anywhere from 7 to 14 days. The traditional wisdom had it that the longer the course of therapy, the better the results. This may not be true, at least according to one study in which treatment for only one day was more effective than the longer course. I still recommend the latter until these observations have been duplicated.

URINARY TRACT
INFECTION

· · · · · · · · ·

A Vaccine Is on the Way

WOMEN ARE MORE PRONE than men to recurrent urinary tract infections because their urinary duct, the urethra, is shorter and more easily reached by bacteria from the anus and the vagina. People with diabetes are especially vulnerable to such infections because they have a weakened immune system and the sugar in their urine provides a good breeding ground for the bug. As a result, between 10 and 15 percent of all women—and at least 20 percent of those who have diabetes—are plagued by this problem.

The main symptom of urinary tract infection is the urge to urinate very frequently, and doing so is accompanied by a painful burning sensation. If the kidneys are also infected, you may have pain in the

251

lower back or abdomen along with fever and occasional nausea and vomiting. The urine is likely to have a strong odor and may be cloudy or blood-tinged. Aside from the discomfort and the inconvenience of running to the john every few minutes (and wearing special diapers in case you don't get there in time), recurrent urinary tract infections can cause further damage. As bacteria move up the urethra, they infect the bladder (cystitis). They then travel to the kidneys, causing a serious condition called pyelonephritis.

When typical symptoms appear, a urine specimen should be sent to the lab for culture to identify the bug that's causing the trouble and to determine the antibiotics to which it's sensitive. The most common organisms responsible for these urinary tract infections belong to the *Escherichia coli* (*E. coli*) family that inhabit the intestinal tract, as well as two sexually transmitted organisms, chlamydia and mycoplasma. (The latter two usually remain in the urethra and do not often spread to the bladder and the kidneys.)

After several days of treatment with the appropriate antibiotic, the symptoms of a urinary tract infection usually clear up. Unfortunately, they often recur a few weeks later—a cycle that tends to be repeated month after month. The frequent use of antibiotics not only eradicates the infecting organism but also destroys harmless bacteria in the vagina that normally prevent the growth of fungus. So frequent cycles of antibiotics leave many women with chronic fungal infections. Other patients develop allergies to the antibiotics, and in many cases the infecting bacteria become antibiotic-resistant. (For some reason not yet understood, the more antibiotics a woman takes, the greater her risk of developing breast cancer—see page 34.)

Although antibiotics are the most effective therapy, there are several steps that you can take to reduce your vulnerability to recurrent urinary tract infections.

- Drink lots of water, cranberry juice, and the juices of other berries.

- Urinate as soon as you feel the urge to do so.

- Wipe from front to back to avoid introducing bacteria from the anus and vagina into the urethra.

- Take showers instead of baths, especially bubble baths.

- Cleanse the genitals before and after intercourse.

- Urinate soon after sex.

HERE'S WHAT'S NEW

Researchers at the University of Wisconsin Medical School in Madison have been trying for several years to develop a vaccine to prevent urinary tract infections. They have succeeded in making one that's delivered via a vaginal suppository. (An earlier, injectable form caused too many side effects.) This vaginal vaccine (Urovac) contains a mixture of heat-killed bacteria from 10 of the most common strains of bacteria responsible for these infections. Delivered via a glycerin-based vaginal suppository, the vaccine stimulates the production of antibodies against these 10 strains of bacteria. It's safe, it can be inserted by the patient, and there are no side effects other than occasional temporary vaginal irritation. A course of treatment consists of one suppository a week for 3 weeks and three boosters at 4-week intervals.

In a recent study of 54 women with a history of at least three urinary tract infections in the previous year, more than half who received a course of the vaccine remained free from infection for at least 6 months. Their average infection-free period was greater than 160 days as compared with 35 days for the group taking only a placebo.

THE BOTTOM LINE

A well-tolerated and effective vaginal vaccine to prevent recurrent urinary tract infections is on the way. Researchers are now conducting large-scale clinical trials that, if successful, will result in the vaccine being marketed and available to everyone in the near future. If you're plagued by such infections, ask your doctor whether such trials are being conducted in your area.

UTERINE
FIBROIDS

· · · · · · · · ·

Pinpointing Relief

ONE IN EVERY FOUR WOMEN in this country develops fibroids as
she grows older. Usually discovered during a routine pelvic exam,
these benign growths of the uterus can be as small as a pinhead or
as large as a melon; most are somewhere in between. Fibroids usually do not cause any symptoms unless they are numerous or huge.
Their presence can be compared to enlargement of the prostate
gland in men in that neither condition leads to cancer, they may or
may not produce symptoms, and there are several treatment options. For uterine fibroids, treatments range from medications to
hysterectomy (removal of the uterus). Fibroids can cause the following symptoms:

- Infertility, miscarriage, premature delivery, and excessive bleeding during labor (in women of childbearing age)
- Menstrual cramping
- Pelvic pain
- Painful intercourse
- Bleeding between periods

When the symptoms are troublesome enough to require treatment, there are several options. The first is nonprescription painkillers such as one of the nonsteroidal anti-inflammatory drugs or acetaminophen. Since excessive estrogen production by the body is believed to cause fibroids and promote the growth of any that already exist, the next step is to use estrogen-blocking drugs such as Lupron (leuprolide), Zoladex (goserelin), and Synarel (nafarelin). Although these medications usually shrink the fibroids, resulting in less pain and bleeding, they cause a "false menopause" in which the periods end, the risk of osteoporosis increases, hot flashes occur, and vaginal tissues become dry.

Danocrine (danazol), a drug that increases the production of the hormone testosterone, is also commonly used to treat troublesome fibroids. Its side effects, such as male hair-growth patterns and a deepening voice, are not acceptable to most women. The main purpose of these medications is to shrink the fibroids before surgery, so the drugs are rarely continued for more than 6 months.

Another treatment is the female hormone progestin (Depo-Provera), which suppresses the formation of estrogen and is particularly effective when the fibroids cause heavy bleeding. However, women with a previous history of or vulnerability to breast cancer should not take progestin.

When none of these medications help—and the fibroids are getting bigger, the pain worsens, the bleeding is heavier, or urination and bowel problems have developed because of the pressure exerted by large fibroids—doctors recommend one of the following:

Hysterectomy. This is the complete surgical removal of the uterus. Although this surgery is done less often these days, 200,000 such operations are still performed every year in the United States. Hysterectomy is major surgery, and it results in infertility.

Myomectomy. During this procedure, the fibroids are removed, leaving the rest of the uterus intact. Newer laparoscopic techniques have made this procedure less invasive, but it, too, is not as frequently used because of other less-intrusive methods.

Endometrial ablation. Laser technology and electrocautery can destroy the lining of the uterus. This is an outpatient procedure that's used when the uterine bleeding is heavy. It results in infertility and removes only very small growths.

Myolysis. With this technique, electricity, heat, or cold is used to interfere with the blood supply to the fibroids so that they shrink and wither away.

Embolization. This is a minimally invasive procedure in which small particles are injected into the blood supply of the fibroids, causing them to shrink. There is no surgery involved, it is not difficult to do, and the results are excellent. This technique is currently favored by gynecologists and their patients, although it may cause some post-procedure pain and fever.

HERE'S WHAT'S NEW

Heating the uterus with focused ultrasound is a promising, new, totally noninvasive approach to the treatment of uterine fibroids. The system is called the ExAblate 2000. Here's how it works. The exact location of the fibroid growth is pinpointed with a combination of magnetic resonance imaging (MRI) and ultrasonography (ultrasound). An ultrasound beam is then delivered at high temperature to the fibroid, cutting off its blood supply. Using MRI to locate the mass makes it possible to direct the ultrasound with great precision so that nothing else in the area is affected.

This is an outpatient procedure that takes about 2 hours, is well tolerated, and thus far has been extremely safe and effective. In the largest study reported to date, only 10 percent of the treated women required pain medication after treatment. The advantages of focused ultrasound treatment over surgery are obvious, and it also appears to cause less pain and fever than does uterine artery embolization. A U.S. advisory panel has urged approval of ExAblate 2000 despite the objections of the National Uterine Fibroids Foundation, a group that recommended further studies for another year. Ongoing trials continue at Harvard-affiliated Brigham and Women's Hospital, the Mayo Clinic, and Johns Hopkins.

THE BOTTOM LINE

Hundreds of thousands of women still undergo hysterectomies for their fibroids. Along with other surgical techniques (and even medication), such treatment now appears to be outdated in many cases in view of the newer, noninvasive techniques for fibroid removal. Among these, the most popular is arterial embolization, in which injected particles occlude the arteries supplying the fibroids and cause them to shrink.

A new technique has recently been introduced: a focused ultrasound treatment that targets the fibroids with pinpoint precision and then delivers enough heat to destroy them. This is completely noninvasive, does not require hospitalization, and is very well tolerated with no significant side effects. I expect the FDA will follow the recommendations of its advisory panel and approve this technique, probably by the time this book is published.

WRINKLES

● ● ● ● ● ● ● ● ●

New Drug Puts Wrinkles to Rest

THERE WAS A TIME when cosmetic surgery was of interest only to women. How times have changed! These days, men too are eager to erase facial wrinkles and other stigmata of aging—both for ego and career enhancement.

Two techniques that are less invasive than the conventional face-lift and tightening procedures have become very popular. The first, and more widely used, is the injection of Botox. A very dilute preparation of botulinum toxin, Botox paralyzes muscles beneath the skin and eliminates frown lines in the forehead. This effect is temporary, and the injections usually need to be repeated at 6-month intervals. The second procedure is the injection of collagen into the skin. Collagen is an important body protein responsible for skin elasticity; its degradation leads to the wrinkles that accompany aging. Collagen removes wrinkles as effectively as Botox, but it also must be done every few months.

HERE'S WHAT'S NEW

Hyaluronic acid is a naturally occurring constituent of connective tissue found throughout the body, including the skin. (It has been used for several years as a treatment for severely osteoarthritic knees. When injected into the affected joint, it sometimes eliminates the need for knee replacement. However, the effectiveness of this therapy is controversial.)

Hyaluronic acid has been called a "key to the Fountain of Youth." Folklore has it that those who consume large amounts in their diets live longer. The FDA has now approved it as yet a third injectable antiwrinkle treatment. It is marketed in this country as Restylane. Hyaluronic acid cushions, lubricates, and keeps the skin "plump." In Europe, it has been used with some success for several years to eliminate wrinkles around the nose and mouth and to improve depressions in the skin caused by scarring from acne or injury.

Like Botox and collagen, hyaluronic acid gradually breaks down and is absorbed after it is injected into the skin, so its treatments also need to be repeated. However, a single augmentation injection with hyaluronic acid usually lasts between 6 and 9 months, somewhat longer than Botox or collagen implants. It can result in increased bruising, swelling, and pain at the site of injection in about 3 percent of cases, but these side effects are mild and clear up in less than 2 weeks.

THE BOTTOM LINE

I'm not sure that there's much to choose from among these three antiwrinkle procedures. If, however, you're considering this approach to improve your appearance, ask the dermatologist who will be administering it to tell you how much it will cost and how frequently you will need to have it done. Remember, such cosmetic therapy is usually not covered by insurance.

INDEX

. . . .

Underscored page references indicate boxed text.